All You Need to
Know About

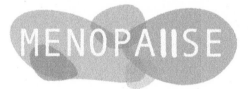

MENOPAUSE

All You Need to Know About

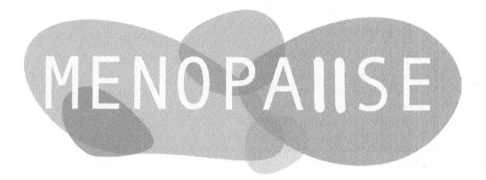

MENOPAUSE

Catherine O'Keeffe

Ireland's Menopause Expert

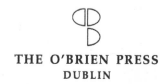

THE O'BRIEN PRESS
DUBLIN

Dedicated to the lovely women of Ireland,
past, present and future.

First published 2023 by
The O'Brien Press Ltd,
12 Terenure Road East, Rathgar,
Dublin 6, D06 HD27, Ireland.
Tel: +353 1 4923333; Fax: +353 1 4922777
E-mail: books@obrien.ie
Website: obrien.ie
The O'Brien Press is a member of Publishing Ireland.

ISBN: 978-1-78849-335-2

8 7 6 5 4 3 2 1
27 26 25 24 23

Printed and bound by Scandbook AB, Sweden.
The paper in this book is produced using pulp from managed forests.

While every effort has been made to ensure the accuracy of the information in this book,
readers should always consult a medical professional or healthcare adviser if seeking medical
advice, diagnosis or treatment: this book is not a substitute. The author and publishers cannot be
held responsible for any risks or issues associated with using or acting upon the information in
this book.

Published in

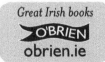

Contents

Introduction

The aim of this book is to be your tool, your friendly guide to navigating what can be a topsy-turvy time. It's to give you the information you need as a best friend would – in a direct and sympathetic way – to help you make informed choices without influencing your decisions: those are yours alone. I want to tell it to you as it is – the good, the bad and the downright ugly aspects. And by the time you close this book, I hope you will feel empowered, informed and, above all, ready to embrace menopause as the inevitable life change that it is.

I have learned so much from the thousands of people I have worked with over the years, and I have always wanted to share that information with more people. How could I condense what I have learned to help others? A book was the answer. I love to see new books on menopause coming out, as they all approach it from a different angle, with a different view. I hope you will find this book different in its own way. The numerous stories I have been humbled to hear, the women who have helped me to learn more, the people who have asked for help for their partners, the questions that have led me to delve further and find answers to share with you – it all culminates in these pages. I am and continue to be a dedicated student of menopause. And it started when I was young – I just didn't know it.

As a child, I spent ample hours lost in books in our local library, which was a stone's throw from our house. In my late twenties, I took a backpack and travelled the world with my faithful journal. If I had thought then that I 'had a book in me', it would have been a tale of the adventures, love and fun on those whirlwind days – or a thriller, even. But a book on menopause was never on my radar.

So how did I end up here, sitting in my garden typing furiously on my laptop about hot flushes, throbbing vaginas and *Wuthering Heights*-style depression? Certainly, that eight-year-old girl in Carnegie Library, Kilkenny, had no notion or knowledge of the term 'menopause'. But our lives bring us on a journey, none of us knowing where we will end up or the pitfalls and joy we will experience along the way.

So here is what I can tell you: menopause is a journey, a deep physiological and psychological rollercoaster ride that will cause anxiety and tears and reveal a depth of character you may never have expected.

I certainly didn't.

If you talked to my friends or family, they would tell you I have always been interested in health and well-being. But I honestly had no idea that my life would take this path. After studying business in college, I started working in investment banking in London. Over the next twenty years, I built a successful career. During this time I also took some time off to travel. Nearly two years later, after many narrow escapes, adventures and new friends, I returned to London two stone heavier and, for the first time in my life, experiencing severe stomach issues. I knew the lunch at a rest stop outside Bangkok was the culprit – a week of horrendous food poisoning was evidence of that – but my stomach did not recover. That was the start of my next journey.

After a series of doctors, scans and tests, I was no better, so I sought any form of natural medicine that could help me to heal. I discovered an amazing naturopath in Greenwich, London, and within three months I was back to normal – all bloating gone and stomach pain a distant memory. I was hooked on all things natural. A few years later, I returned to college and studied natural medicine while continuing to work in investment banking – two polar-opposite worlds. I got married, continued to climb the corporate ladder, had three boys and then hit a wall. One evening, I came home after an exhausting day at work. All I wanted to do was get the boys to bed and veg out in front of the TV. Unfortunately, I'd completely forgotten we had friends calling over. Instead of being excited, I dreaded their arrival as I rushed to get the house ready and whip a meal together. The pressure was unreal. Even though I hadn't seen our friends in ages, I didn't enjoy a single moment from that evening. That's when I knew my life had to change. Accompanied constantly by a Blackberry (remember those?), never switching off, working hard, returning home each day to my second job, it was constant juggling. I felt burnt out; I felt stuck, hemmed in – I desperately wanted a change. On top of everything, perimenopause had started.

My wake-up call came a month later, when I was sitting in a restaurant in Copenhagen with my college friends. It was November, and we were all dressed up for a night out – ready and rearing to go! Sheer panic ensued when, during the main course, I felt a deluge of blood leaving my body. My head spun. Here I was with some of my closest friends and I couldn't even get the words out to explain what was happening. I let my napkin fall to the ground so I could bend over and get some sense of how bad things were. Not a pleasant sight. All I could see was blood on my seat. I didn't dare go to the toilet for fear of people seeing my blood-soaked clothes. The chair was ruined. I survived dessert and got through the meal. On leaving, I had to tie my jacket around my waist – I was so cold stepping out into the Copenhagen winter and still in shock about what had happened.

The killer was that I knew I was fine. On returning home, I booked a GP appointment and had another scan – no issues whatsoever. It was one of those somewhat rare occurrences of perimenopause – my infamous 'flooding' incident.

I did acupuncture, and within two cycles my periods were back to normal. But I knew I was beginning perimenopause, so I started to find out as much as I could about what was happening and how I could support myself. I started running – anyone who knew me from my school days will know I used every monthly period I had to escape PE classes! It was the one subject I always failed. But a friend was doing Couch to 5K and asked me to join, and I took to it like a duck to water. I loved the feel-good hormone release I got after each session. Today it is still my go-to for managing daily stress – it's my mental-health break. I also delved into as much health research as possible, investigating periods, moods, bloating, anxiety, loss of confidence, libido – you name it. After Copenhagen, I wanted to be fully prepared for anything that menopause was going to throw at me!

And juggling work and a busy home life became more of a struggle with the onset of perimenopause. I vividly recall one day being in a boardroom, ready to present to management from New York. As a director in investment banking, meetings and presentations were a regular thing – no sweat on that front. We had visiting executives, our own management team, myself and one other uninvited, unexpected guest: my perimenopause. Just minutes into the presentation, every piece of information I was hoping to deliver flew out of my head, which instead filled with brain fog, memory loss and embarrassment. Anxiety and perimenopause were in collision. I wanted the ground to open up. Menopause, though, was here to stay. My stomach still turns over as I recall that day. It left a big dent in my confidence and a spike in my frustration with what was happening to my body.

To this day, I can remember the view out that window, the window that my knowledge of specifics flew right out of. It had never, in all my career, happened to me before, yet there I sat, feeling my brain devoid of all sense and information. If you have been in that seat for even a minute, you will know how it feels. And, since then, there have been many more moments like that, but I learned from each one along the way and armed myself with the knowledge I needed to navigate my own menopause and work.

I had learned a lot about health and well-being over the years, but when I started to concentrate on women's health and menopause it became all-encompassing and intriguing – for personal reasons and also because of the taboo and silence around it in Ireland. I felt a pull toward a new career and left the world of investment banking behind. The gap in knowledge that existed across society was very evident. This spurred me on and fuelled my passion – I started travelling around Ireland and talking to packed rooms of women about menopause and all it entails. I mean, really talking …

I have been told on many occasions that I opened the doors to taboo subjects – things women were embarrassed to discuss even with those closest to them. I've seen pure relief when women realised they were not going mad, that it was, in fact, their hormones and the trials of menopause making them feel as they did. On several occasions, women have cried with me with relief, which is humbling and touching. I vividly remember a brave woman at one of my talks who had to sit on an inflatable ring cushion because she was experiencing such severe vaginal dryness and pain in her pelvic area. She had been told that this was her life now and that intimacy would no longer feature. It was harrowing. This should not be the case – women should be fully supported in the medical system of the country they live in and have access to knowledge about their symptoms.

While I love and have studied complementary medicine, and find it very helpful, I am also aware of the necessity of all treatment forms when it comes to menopause. HRT (hormone replacement therapy) has received very bad press over the years, and it is an area I have worked extensively on – ensuring women have accurate knowledge of this treatment and all other options they can pursue. Too often I talk with women who are prescribed antidepressants that, for the most part, are not what is required: the hormonal change is what needs to be addressed. Educating women on their choices ensures they can seek and demand the right treatment – this starts with talking more about menopause. We are certainly making great progress in this, in Ireland and globally, but there is still much to do. So many women feel lonely and isolated in these years. This should not be the case. Medical and therapeutic professionals also need basic education and training in menopause that continues throughout their career. Women need to feel supported. So we need to open up this conversation – for women, for families and for workplaces.

All women work – whether outside the home or at home, every woman works on a daily basis. Managing your menopause symptoms while doing so can pose additional challenges. Every role comes with its own stresses, and stress is a major contributing factor (along with those good old hormones leaving us) to many menopause symptoms. And part of that stress can come from your dual roles – the worker bee and the menopausal bee. The symptoms you experience may be the same as other people's, but the impact they have on you and your work will differ. The differences can be based on your environment, your job, your internal coping mechanisms and much more. Discussions are happening in the workplace on this topic, and I applaud those forward-thinking employers who have opened the doors to the conversation. To date, I have spoken to thousands of employees at the invitation of their employers, and I have seen at first hand the positive impact it has on women: they feel happier in their jobs, they feel supported and they feel empowered, because they are being listened to by their employers.

My work today is different from my days in the corporate world, but establishing a business and being an entrepreneur comes with its own set of challenges, and what I have learned most is that – while it never feels like work to me because helping and inspiring people in relation to menopause is my passion – the journey you go on when building your own business is a personal one of ongoing self-discovery. And menopause is this too, so perhaps now, for me, the 'twain' are meeting in a purposeful way in the culmination of what I know can be the most rewarding chapter in a woman's life.

When I started perimenopause, I knew the general symptoms we all talk about – hot flushes, night sweats and so on – but I didn't know half of what I know now about pelvic dysfunction, vaginal atrophy, depression and so much more. I have learned so much – I am learning more every day. And now it's time to get this information out to as many people as possible – not just to women, but to men too: we all know someone in menopause right this minute.

Daily, I am learning from personal research and study, but it's from the many lovely women I work and talk with that I learn the most. From face-to-face chats, live interviews on social media, video calls from cowsheds, cars, toilets, beaches, attics and the kitchen table – all these interactions with thousands of women have laid the foundations for this book. This has culminated with the launch of the Menopause Success Summit, where bringing women together in bigger numbers is shattering the taboo of menopause and allowing them to hear first-hand from experts on all aspects of menopause and to meet fellow warriors on the same journey, alleviating any feelings of isolation and loneliness that can come with menopause.

Menopause may impact all ages and all genders. Trans men, trans women, non-binary people and genderfluid people can also experience menopause or symptoms of menopause. As gender is a spectrum, the individual experience must be listened to. Throughout this book, you will see the term *woman* mainly used, as this reflects the people with whom I have worked to date. This is not in any way to lessen the impact on others.

So, I hope you, the reader, are sitting with your cuppa, relaxed and open to receiving the information in this book. I am not a medical doctor: I am a woman on a mission to get information about the menopause out there. I'm here to help you understand what is happening and provide answers to the questions you have.

This book is designed for you to be able to dip into, so each chapter can be read in isolation. With menopause, symptoms may change from month to month – I have worked with women who have had hot flushes to beat the band for years that then stop, only to be replaced by brain fog or another symptom. This book will provide informed, factual advice on the steps you can take as different symptoms appear.

The book is split into sections to make navigating large subjects easier. Part 1 tells you all about menopause – what it really is and what it isn't, and what if it comes early. Part 2 jumps into the symptoms of menopause and gives you tips for how to address them, including in the workplace. Part 3 covers all the options, from HRT to acupuncture to CBT (cognitive behavioural therapy), that can help you. Part 4 looks at the 6 Ms, my guiding principles to help you thrive through these years, as I firmly believe that, once you get a handle on your symptoms, you can flourish in this chapter of your life. Part 5 includes a chapter for your partner and thoughts on how we can continue to break the menopause taboo in a diverse, inclusive way.

There is also a detailed references and resources section, which I encourage you to make use of, listing the research materials I have used and invaluable websites to explore as you navigate your journey through menopause.

So, right now, maybe jump straight to that symptom that's causing you the most hassle – that's my best-friend's advice to you. And when you feel empowered to handle that symptom with the practical advice given, please do come back here to the very beginning and read in more detail about the what, the why and the how of menopause.

Part 1: What's It All About?

1

Perimenopause and menopause

The menopause journey is different for every single person, and that can make it unknown territory. When we understand what may happen, it helps reduce the fear and anxiety that can arise around this inevitable life stage. A key starting point is knowing what menopause is and why it happens.

I have had numerous conversations over the years with clients who are puzzled as to what is happening in their bodies – why, all of a sudden, intense emotions are a daily feature of life, why the thought of going out with friends makes them anxious or why they feel a churning belly before regular daily events. With not a hot flush in sight, the subtle and not-so-subtle changes that signal the start of perimenopause can take women by surprise. It's sneaky, perimenopause. From sometimes slight changes in the early days, it can build to a crescendo with the arrival of the first typical symptoms – perhaps an intense hot flush or a drenching night sweat – leaving you wondering what's happening to your body.

It's normal, it's menopause, it's inevitable.

And it doesn't just happen to humans – female whales and giraffes also experience menopause, albeit in a very different ecosystem. Whales stop reproducing in their thirties and forties and live in a non-productive state for many years after, mirroring the human experience of menopause, and becoming a wise matriarch within the pod. Giraffes spend 30 per cent of their lives post-menopause.

Right now, more than one billion women are experiencing menopause. So what is it all about and where does it come from?

MENOPAUSE IN HISTORY

If we refer back to ancient Greek and Chinese writings we can find mentions of menstruation and references to menopause. As far back as the fourth century BCE, Aristotle indicated that the average age of menopause was fifty. In the second century BCE, the Chinese made great progress in the study of endocrinology (understanding hormones) and are arguably its founders. They separated sex and pituitary hormones from human urine and used the output to treat ailments ranging from dysmenorrhea to impotence (in ways, a very early form of HRT). Hildegard of Bingen, a twelfth-century nun, wrote about the uterus folding and contracting and periods stopping between fifty and sixty years of age.

On a darker note, in the Salem witch trials of 1692 thirteen of the women accused were in the menopause age range. And we can thank the Victorians for turning menopause into a mental illness and sending many women to institutions to help with their 'hysteria'.

Menopause has a complex and often dark history.

The actual first use of the word 'menopause' was in 1821 by French doctor Charles de Gardanne, who had previously coined it 'menespausie'. 'Menes' is the Greek root for month and 'pausie' means cessation.

Historical references before and up to that point often referred to menopause as the 'climacteric', 'change', 'cessation' or 'critical age'. It was also known as 'the dodging time', which I like for its lightness.

Medically, menopause is defined as when you have had twelve months without a period, but the word is also used more generally to encompass the time leading up to that anniversary – the whole process.

STAGES OF A NATURAL MENSTRUAL CYCLE

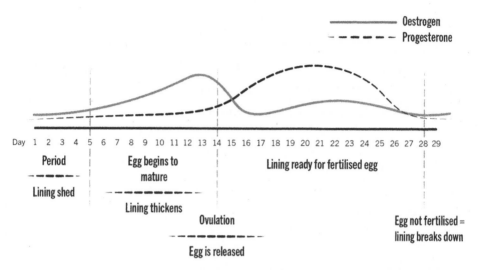

If life is a rollercoaster, for many women, perimenopause is Alton Towers. It all starts with your monthly hormonal rollercoaster: your menstrual cycle. The two are inextricably linked. When we are born, we are already on a planned journey to menopause (early menopause is an exception). The route is in the sat nav, ready to go. Your menstrual cycle is the key to understanding the importance of menopause hormones and the journey you will go on.

Days 1–5: Your period starts. Prior to this, levels of progesterone and oestrogen (big players in menopause) will have dropped and triggered the shedding of the uterine lining, resulting in your period. The fall in oestrogen and also inhibin creates an increase in FSH (follicle-stimulating hormone). FSH is made in the pituitary gland and communicates with your ovaries. Now, FSH gets to work and sends a message to the ovaries for the immature follicles to start developing. Your period can last three to eight days, with five being the average. Oestrogen production begins to increase.

Days 5–14: Generally, one follicle will respond to the messages from the pituitary gland. This now-maturing follicle starts to produce oestrogen and inhibin in large quantities. This will cause FSH, which reaches its highest level just before the egg is released, to fall. The increase in oestrogen will also stimulate the uterine lining to thicken in preparation for a fertilised egg.

Days 14–25: Oestrogen levels peak, telling the pituitary gland to release luteinising hormone (LH). The LH increase tells the developing follicle to release the egg from the ovaries, and it begins its adventure down the fallopian tube to the uterus. Progesterone production begins to increase.

Days 25–28: Now the mature follicle begins to produce progesterone. This works alongside oestrogen to prepare the lining of the womb to receive an egg. If there is no fertilised egg, the two key hormones drop, the lining sheds and your period starts.

This is based on the average cycle, but your menstrual cycle can go anywhere from twenty-one to thirty-five days – like menopause, it is unique to you. Your menstrual cycle can be seen as your fifth vital sign and brings with it health-restoring properties, so we want to keep our cycles going naturally for as long as possible. (If you are on the contraceptive pill, you don't have a menstrual period but a withdrawal bleed.) You can also see how FSH fluctuates throughout the cycle – this is why it is not used as a key indicator of menopause.

YOUR CYCLE MATTERS AND EGGS MATTER

Two key parts of the menstrual cycle are the ovaries and follicles. Before birth, the female ovaries already store what are called dormant follicles – eggs waiting to mature (these are called your ovarian reserve). On average, there are one to two million of these follicles at birth. When a girl reaches adolescence, she has between 300,000 and 500,000 eggs; once she begins menstruating, ovulation occurs once a month, releasing mature follicles.

Menopause is when that store of follicles is depleted (you have gone from millions of eggs to just a few thousand). There are no more left to ovulate each month, and this has an effect on hormones, as the menstrual cycle is reliant on the monthly release of an egg.

The follicles are a key source of oestrogen, so when the cycle stops, it leads to a sharp decline in oestrogen production. In the pre-menopause years, the average body will produce 250 to 300 micrograms of oestrogen daily. Post-menopause, this dips to 20 micrograms. This decline in oestrogen will have an impact for many women.

Hormones are chemical messengers that control the functioning of our bodies. Perimenopause is when they truly demonstrate how powerful they are. The three key hormones involved – oestrogen, progesterone and testosterone – fluctuate and gradually decline through these years.

THE STAGES OF MENOPAUSE

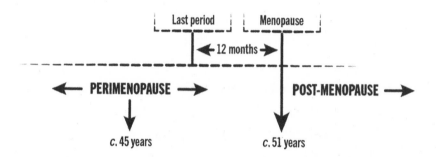

Perimenopause is the start of the hormonal changes, the beginning stage for menopause (the culminating event). For many, progesterone is the hormone that starts to get 'wobbly' first, and this is when the psychological symptoms of menopause often start to show themselves – changing moods, anxiety, loss of confidence and more. At this stage, progesterone lowers while oestrogen can be higher and dominant. Your periods can still be regular or may change by a few days and/or become lighter or heavier. This isn't just over weeks or months: it's over years. The average age perimenopause starts at is forty-five. (Perimenopause may only apply to natural menopause – it will not be experienced if menopause is induced, in which case you bypass it and go straight into full-blown menopause, unless you are already on the perimenopause journey.)

Do you remember the rollercoaster of hormones you felt at fourteen? The changing moods, the constant need to eat, the skin changes, the body changes of puberty? Menopause is reverse puberty, with the different hormones colliding and declining in the latter years.

Perimenopause can be broken down into four key stages:

1. **Very early or subtle perimenopause:** cycle length can be the same or change slightly. Many women report seeing the start or return of PMT-like symptoms or experiencing night sweats before and during their period. You may start to feel 'different', possibly more anxious or just not yourself. You may also start to notice that you can go from zero to a hundred in nanoseconds, and feelings of rage are very common – that 'flying off the handle' experience. Progesterone dips and oestrogen will be higher.

2. **The irregular-periods or early perimenopause years:** cycle length and flow now change in a noticeable way. Oestrogen remains high but fluctuates wildly. Progesterone continues to dip and changes may be experienced in testosterone levels also. Physical symptoms start to become more obvious.

3. **The skipping years or later perimenopause:** the duration between cycles becomes longer (generally three to six months). The physical symptoms, like brain fog, hot flushes, night sweats and vaginal atrophy, may be heightened. Oestrogen and progesterone are both now low, possibly testosterone too.

4. **Edging close to menopause:** hot flushes, night sweats and vaginal dryness will be very common now for many.

Menopause is the next chapter after perimenopause, and it is like an anniversary of sorts: it's the mark of twelve months without a monthly cycle. Is that it then

– no more periods? Generally, it is, but sometimes there may be a final period or two that insist on saying goodbye before they fully stop. The average age for menopause is fifty-one. This varies based on geographical location and ethnicity – for example, the average age in Africa is forty-eight and in the US it's fifty.

Then it's **post-menopause**. This isn't a defined chapter but the rest of a person's life. Also, symptoms can, and will for many, continue into the post-menopause years. Menopause does not equate to the end of symptoms. The ways to support yourself described throughout the book also apply to post-menopause unless otherwise stated.

TYPES OF MENOPAUSE

While the majority of women will experience natural menopause, other forms can also occur. Earlier forms are when menopause occurs before the average age of fifty-one. Premature ovarian insufficiency (POI) means menopause before the age of forty, and early menopause is when menopause itself happens between age forty and forty-five. Early menopause can also be due to surgery or medication. (See Chapter 2 for further discussion.) If you experience early menopause for medical or surgical reasons, you may bypass the perimenopause stage and go straight into menopause – this is why these experiences are often referred to as 'cliff-edge' menopause.

Andropause is a male form of menopause, with symptoms resulting from the testosterone decline that comes with age. Research to date tells us it impacts 30 per cent of men, while all women will go through menopause.

HOW MENOPAUSE BEGINS

Think about your hormones like a jigsaw puzzle: every part has its place. Each hormone is a chemical messenger that moves around your body looking for where it fits into the puzzle – for its receptor.

Understanding the three main hormones involved in menopause (progesterone, oestrogen and testosterone) and how they interact can be very helpful.

Progesterone

Let's start with progesterone, the soothing hormone, the mood and sleep supporter, the yin to oestrogen's yang, its partner in the hormonal dance. It is made in the ovaries, goes out of balance in perimenopause and tends to be the hormone that starts its gradual decline the earliest. We think of it as the essential hormone for fertility, and the name itself means 'promoting gestation', but it does more. It is a key part of bone health (for bone formation) and also plays a part in the prevention of uterine cancer. When we delve into HRT, you will hear more about this (see Chapter 14). Progesterone is also known for its impact on mood and sleep. It creates allopregnanolone, which has a calming influence on the receptors in your brain.

The key benefits of progesterone are that it:

- Thins the uterine lining
- Reduces anxiety
- Induces sleep
- Has anti-inflammatory properties
- Builds bones
- Protects the heart
- Impacts metabolic rate

PROGESTERONE TOO LOW	PROGESTERONE TOO HIGH
Memory issues	Breast tenderness
Weight gain	Bloating
Low libido	Mood swings
PMT symptoms	Dizziness
Mood swings	
Cyclical headaches	
Heavy periods	

In perimenopause, progesterone levels start to decline, and its balance with oestrogen can go out of kilter – you may now have more oestrogen than before in your body. This imbalance will trigger symptoms like mood changes, breast tenderness, headaches, sleep issues and heavy periods. It is only after your final period that you reach a state of low hormones. Prior to that, it is all about fluctuation.

Oestrogen

This is the queen bee of hormones – the zest that sparks within every woman. But sometimes it can get too sparky, too high, and during perimenopause it may be the highest it has ever been. Erratic is the best word to describe oestrogen, especially in the early perimenopause years.

The reduction in oestrogen levels would be fine if oestrogen was just responsible for egg production, but that's not the case. Oestrogen affects nearly every cell in our bodies, which is why we experience symptoms and also why no two women will experience menopause in the same way. One person might get hot flushes; another might never get them but might suffer from anxiety or palpitations.

There are four types of oestrogen: 17b oestradiol, oestrone, oestriol and oestetrol:

- 17b oestradiol is the strongest form of oestrogen. It peaks in pre-menopause then crashes post-menopause. The amount of oestrogen moving through the body changes throughout the monthly cycle and tends to peak right before ovulation. Oestradiol has a function in protecting the heart, brain and bones, but it also plays a role in over three hundred other processes within the body.
- Oestrone, produced by the adrenal glands and fatty tissue, is the key form of oestrogen made in the body in the post-menopause years. It has much weaker biological activity than oestradiol and doesn't pack the same punch.
- Oestriol levels are generally very low, but during pregnancy it is made in much higher amounts by the placenta. Oestriol levels increase throughout pregnancy and are highest just before birth. This is the form you will see

later being used for vaginal and urinary symptoms of menopause.

• Oestetrol is made by the developing foetus during pregnancy. Clinical trials are being performed to look at this form of oestrogen as a possible support for menopause symptoms.

Oestrogen can sometimes be too high. This is generally in the early perimenopause years and can result in heavy periods, as oestrogen causes the endometrial lining to thicken – especially if your body is not producing enough progesterone to balance this out.

As you enter the late perimenopause stage, oestrogen is on the decline, and the high fluctuations will have reduced. This is when you may see the genitourinary symptoms of menopause taking centre stage and the very physical symptoms vying for their time in the limelight.

Your ovaries will completely stop producing progesterone in menopause, but oestrogen can still be produced in other areas of the body. As egg production is no longer required in menopause, oestrogen is then produced in areas like the skin and adrenal glands.

OESTROGEN TOO LOW	OESTROGEN TOO HIGH
Hot flushes, nights sweats	Change in sleep
Headaches	Weight gain
Mood swings	Hair loss
Vaginal dryness	Headaches
Mucous membrane thinning	Memory issues
Urinary incontinence	Appetite changes

Testosterone

Testosterone is often thought of as the male hormone, but women need it too. Surprisingly, women produce three times as much testosterone as oestrogen before the menopause.

Testosterone is primarily made in two locations and split equally between them – 25 per cent in the ovaries, both in the follicle and also in the ovary itself, and 25 per cent in the adrenal glands (the small glands near your kidneys). The remaining 50 per cent is made throughout the body in the fatty tissue.

Because testosterone is not mainly produced by the ovaries, it does not experience the same reduction in levels that oestrogen does after menopause. But as we get older, testosterone declines, with the result that your libido drops, and when you do have sex, it may not be as pleasurable as it used to be. Currently, testosterone is medically prescribed for low libido.

Testosterone is important for bone strength, heart health, cognitive performance, energy levels and general feelings of well-being. But some women may have a time when testosterone becomes dominant and they can have symptoms like acne, excess hair growth and even a deepening voice (very rare).

Loss of testosterone is particularly challenging after surgical menopause, as the levels fall by more than 50 per cent. Those with POI and medical menopause will also experience significant loss of testosterone.

TESTOSTERONE TOO LOW	TESTOSTERONE TOO HIGH
Muscle loss	Excess body hair
Weight gain	Acne
Mood swings	Increased muscle mass
Sexual dysfunction/loss of libido	Changes in body shape
	Irregular periods

Other important players

Gonadotropin-releasing hormone (GnRH): Have you ever watched the *Minions* movie? Their leader is Gru, and whatever Gru says, his minions follow suit. This is what GnRH is to your body – it's Gru. The hypothalamus in your brain releases this essential ingredient. It sends a message to the pituitary gland that triggers your FSH and LH (more on those below) into action. As we age, GnRH loses its sharpness – messages may not be sent as effectively and that starts a chain reaction with the other hormones.

Follicle-stimulating hormone (FSH): This is made by the brain and sends messages to the ovaries to make oestrogen, promoting the growth and development of ovarian follicles. Its levels can fluctuate – in the early perimenopause years, you may experience high FSH on an infrequent basis, with the levels becoming higher as you are closer to menopause.

DHEA (dehydroepiandrosterone): This is not a superstar in its own right, but its power comes from the fact that it converts into other hormones, primarily oestrogen and testosterone. The ovaries can make a small amount, but it is mainly made in your adrenal glands from cholesterol. Once you hit post-menopause, it is the only producer of testosterone and oestrogen. It is a part of the androgen family.

Luteinising hormone (LH): Produced by the pituitary gland, this mighty hormone is responsible for the release of an egg from the ovaries and stimulates the ovaries to produce oestrogen and progesterone.

Leptin: This hormone regulates hunger and metabolism and helps our bodies adjust how we burn fat.

Insulin: Made in the pancreas, this drives glucose into our cells to be used as fuel (energy) and deposits fat. (For more, see Chapter 10.)

Thyroid: This essential gland plays a big role in metabolism and growth and helps regulate many functions in your body. It is associated with energy, weight and mood. It also regulates how the body uses energy and produces heat – many people with thyroid issues feel the cold more. When it is healthy, your thyroid produces hormones (TSH, T4, T3 and others) in the right balance so you feel energetic, don't experience brain fog and feel good. Low thyroid (also known as hypothyroid) results in feelings of sluggishness and poor memory. Many women misinterpret these feelings as menopause or age – hence, having annual blood tests is a good idea. Hyperthyroid (also known as an overactive thyroid) is less common; symptoms are heart palpitations, shortness of breath and weight loss. One in eight women will have a thyroid issue at some stage in their life.

Cortisol: This hormone is just as important as oestrogen and progesterone, as it has a huge impact on women's lives. Cortisol is produced by the adrenal glands and is an essential aspect of your body's fight-or-flight reaction. Cortisol demands our respect: much of your optimum health in menopause and in the future is reliant on this hormone. Too much cortisol causes you to feel tired but 'wired' – your mind and body just can't settle. Too little cortisol makes you feel drained, like a car running on empty. (For more, see Chapter 4.)

Sex hormone binding globulin (SHBG): The liver produces this protein, which binds to sex hormones (oestrogen and testosterone) in both men and women. It regulates how much testosterone your body tissues can use. The amount of SHBG in your blood varies depending on your gender and age. Obesity, liver illness and hyperthyroidism are some conditions that might cause it to change.

FREQUENTLY ASKED QUESTIONS

Though every woman's journey through menopause is different, people often have the same questions. Here are some of the commonest ones I'm asked about menopause.

Why does menopause age differ?

The vast majority of women worldwide will enter menopause aged fifty to fifty-two years. The variations are small and can differ based on geographical location and ethnic background.

Does it really matter what age it happens to you?

It definitely does. As we will see with the early forms of menopause, there can be long-term health consequences that need to be addressed (see Chapter 2). Menopause occurring later than age fifty-four can be associated with an increased risk of endometrial and breast cancer.

What can impact age of menopause?

One of the myths I often hear is that the age you got your first period is indicative of when you will start menopause. Starting your periods earlier does not mean you will automatically start menopause earlier. Research to date on this has not been conclusive.

If your mother had an early menopause or late menopause, studies show you could have a similar experience. Smoking can trigger earlier menopause by two years. Toxins in your environment – pesticides, plastics, chemicals – can also have an impact. A history of heavy periods and a lowered immune system may influence your experience of menopause too, as will your general health – underlying health conditions may result in entering menopause earlier.

I hear about millions of symptoms. How tough is this going to be?

Let's not get ahead of ourselves – there is light at the end of the tunnel!

The facts are that 25 per cent of women will go through menopause reporting no symptoms at all – you could be one of the lucky ones! And 25 per cent will experience severe symptoms, with the balance falling in between, with mild to moderate symptoms.

Remember, you are on your own unique and personal journey through these years, and being able to make informed choices around the supports *you* need is the key. Think of the perimenopause years as navigating the high seas – you are the ship in seas that can be calm (all is well) then quickly change to stormy (symptoms). The better the condition the ship is in, the better your chances of a smooth journey through any choppy waters that arise.

Can a blood test tell me I am in perimenopause?

Yes and no. In perimenopause, as the hormones are constantly changing, symptoms are the best indicator of what is happening within the body. Blood tests are great for checking overall health and ruling out any other underlying health conditions like anaemia (low iron) and thyroid imbalance – these two, in particular, can show symptoms very similar to menopause. The key marker medical professionals use for determining that menopause has happened is the FSH level, mentioned previously. However, these levels can fluctuate, and this is why looking at symptoms is so important. You can be in full-blown perimenopause and your bloods may not reflect it – but the tsunami of symptoms will! Remember, too, our hormone levels are changing hourly and daily.

Aside from ruling out other conditions, blood tests are an effective way of monitoring how HRT treatment is working – a blood test can show oestrogen levels being absorbed into the bloodstream. This tends to be more accurate for transdermal options (absorbed through the skin) than oral HRT (see Chapter 14 for more).

If you are having a blood test to look at hormone levels, three key ones will be taken into account – oestradiol, testosterone and SHBG.

My periods are still regular. How do I know if I am in perimenopause?

You can still have regular periods and be in the throes of perimenopause. Generally, as you get closer to menopause the cycles tend to become more erratic. So a woman who starts to go over fifty-five to sixty days between cycles is most likely in the latter phase of her perimenopause years. Here the final cycle might be three years away or less.

When it comes to knowing if you are in perimenopause, you need to look at the symptoms in their entirety and understand what your body is telling you.

I am on the pill. How do I know where I am during these years?

When you're on the pill, you can't tell if you've entered menopause. This is because hormonal contraception can alter your menstrual cycle. If you take the combined pill, you will get monthly period-like bleeding (withdrawal bleeds) for as long as you take it. If you're on a progestogen-only pill, your periods may become erratic or cease completely for as long as you're on it. Menopausal symptoms like hot flushes and night sweats may be masked or controlled by the combined tablet. These characteristics can make determining menopause difficult. If a woman is on the combination pill, the FSH test is likewise not a reliable indicator that ovulation has ended. For women over fifty who are on a progestogen-only pill, it can be a useful guide.

GETTING MENOPAUSE READY

So now you know about menopause and the important hormones involved, as well as why knowing your menstrual cycle and the hormones that affect you at each stage is crucial to your awareness and empowerment.

This is the time you should get a journal going, start tracking where your body is at and prepare to future-proof yourself through your menopause into those later years.

Here are the top things to track on a monthly basis:

- Your cycle dates.
- Period flow – any changes. Is it heavier? Lighter?
- Any new symptoms, and if so, when they are happening – in early perimenopause it can be close to your period being due.
- What triggers your symptoms?
- How you are feeling? Keep a close eye on your mental health.

* * *

How your perimenopause and menopause years will play out for you cannot be predicted, but being ready and having all the information at hand, knowing where you can get the right help and advice to set yourself up for success in these years, will empower and comfort you.

2

When menopause comes early

When I started studying and researching menopause I was struck by the many forms of early menopause and by premature ovarian insufficiency (POI) in particular. At the time, I struggled to find any information in Ireland and luckily I came upon the Daisy Network, a UK-based charity. Since then, I have spoken with women who started to experience hot flushes as young as twelve years old.

This chapter is about all forms of early menopause – from POI to surgical and medical menopause. When menopause comes early it is a very challenging experience, and it is imperative to have the right supports and knowledge at your fingertips as you navigate this terrain.

PREMATURE OVARIAN INSUFFICIENCY

The terms 'premature ovarian insufficiency' and 'premature menopause' both relate to the same form of menopause, which we'll refer to as POI here.

The European Society of Human Reproduction and Embryology (ESHRE) defines POI as 'a clinical syndrome defined by loss of ovarian activity before the age of 40 years characterised by menstrual disturbance (amenorrhea or oligomenorrhea) with raised gonadotrophins and low oestradiol'.

Basically, it means the ovaries aren't working as they should or they work sporadically. Two key things happen: the ovaries stop producing eggs; and the ovaries cannot produce the essential hormones (oestrogen and progesterone). This low hormone level causes menopause symptoms to appear. The long-term implications are crucial to understand, as many women affected by POI will lose this essential hormone supply years before the average woman, which will impact bone, heart and brain health.

When you are born, your eggs are already in your ovaries. Most women are born with one to two million eggs, but if you have a smaller number at birth or the egg count falls more quickly then you may develop POI.

Recent studies estimate that POI affects:

- 1 in 100 women under forty
- 1 in 1,000 women under thirty
- 1 in 10,000 women under twenty

Why does it happen?

About 90 per cent of POI cases occur for unknown (idiopathic) reasons, so clearly more research is needed. The other reasons for POI are:

- **Autoimmune disease** – roughly 5 per cent of cases are linked to such diseases, where the immune system attacks the body. There are numerous autoimmune conditions, including Hashimoto's disease, Addison's disease, lupus, rheumatoid arthritis and type 1 diabetes. If you have any of these conditions, you should ask your doctor or consultant to check for POI also.
- **Genetics** – generally an abnormality involving the X (female) chromo-some; 10–15 per cent will have a mother or sister who also has POI.
- **Infection** – POI has been reported as sometimes occurring after a serious infection like mumps, tuberculosis or malaria, and 13 per cent of HIV patients will be diagnosed with POI.
- **Surgery** – when the ovaries are removed before the age of forty (due to ovarian cancer, ovarian cysts, endometriosis or other conditions), it will result in POI.

- **Medical treatment** – some cancer treatments like chemotherapy or radiotherapy may cause temporary or permanent damage to the ovaries, which again will cause POI.
- **Polycystic ovary syndrome (PCOS)** – research is ongoing but when a woman has PCOS there may be a 3 to 4 per cent risk of POI.

How is it diagnosed?

I have seen first-hand how difficult it is to get a diagnosis and find the right help. I believe as we increase awareness among doctors and all people we will see more accurate reporting of girls and women impacted by POI.

The first red flag is when you miss three or more periods consecutively and you are under forty years of age. An initial conversation with your doctor should rule out sudden weight loss, thyroid imbalance, PCOS and pregnancy. If these are clear then you should have more detailed blood work. These tests should include the following:

- **FSH level** – if this is over twenty-four, menopause is close to happening or has happened.
- **Luteinising hormone (LH)** – high LH levels indicate the follicles are not functioning normally.
- **Prolactin (a hormone produced in the brain by the pituitary gland)** – higher than normal levels can cause irregular periods and infertility.
- **Oestradiol** – this will be low with POI.
- **Testosterone** – many with POI have lower levels of testosterone compared with other women their age.

Depending on the results, a repeat blood test may need to be taken after four weeks. A scan can be helpful to see if there is anything physically wrong with the ovaries or uterus. This can also see how many follicles are in the ovaries. If POI is confirmed, one of the next important steps is a DXA scan (see Chapter 7).

Additional testing your doctor may recommend

- **Diabetes** – due to the connection with autoimmune illness it is important to investigate for diabetes.
- **Adrenal antibodies** – checking the health of the adrenal glands is another key step.
- **Hypoparathyroidism** – this is not as straightforward as thyroid imbalance and has been associated with POI.
- **HIV** – POI is common among people with HIV.

I was diagnosed with POI aged twenty-five in June 2020. I had not had a period in the six months leading to my diagnosis. I did not have any menopause symptoms other than that my periods stopped. A number of tests were undertaken and no known cause has been identified for my early menopause. I have been quite lucky in that I have not had any drastic symptoms. However, for me, I noticed I had dry eyes, vaginal dryness and mood swings. The most difficult thing for me during this time has been dealing with the effect on my fertility options. Unfortunately, two months after my diagnosis I had some tests and scans which showed no follicles in either ovary. Therefore, my only option is donor-egg IVF if I would like to carry a baby. I started HRT three months after my diagnosis and have changed from oral only to transdermal (patches) and progesterone (as I have an intact womb). This works for me and I've got used to changes and tweaks to my dose to reduce any sensitivity. Throughout this process, I have accessed therapy for feelings of grieving for the loss of my fertility. I found that I was losing control of where I wanted to be on this journey. With the right hormone balance, responding well to HRT, Pilates and therapy, I've learnt to control any problem by controlling how I react to it. I feel this will help me when I experience any other menopause symptoms throughout my POI journey. I've made some lifestyle changes including diet, sleep, routine, exercise, water and vitamins. To my fellow POI ladies – you got this!

– Dani

What needs to happen in caring for someone with POI?

The long-term complications of POI include reduced bone mineral density, resulting in an increased risk of developing osteoporosis and fractures, increased risk of cardiovascular disease and reduced cognition. These risks increase the longer a woman has POI. HRT or a contraceptive containing oestrogen is a key step in the POI journey. It is very important to replace the oestrogen that the body is not producing, and either option will do that.

The standard rules outlined in Chapter 14 will apply here, but usually a higher dose of HRT is required. Generally, HRT is recommended until a woman reaches the natural age of menopause, but this is an individual and personal choice.

Treatment of POI in Ireland can be supported by referral from your GP to a complex menopause clinic. Many women with POI may not be taking HRT or may not be informed about HRT. This is an essential first step for anyone diagnosed with POI. In addition, you may be referred to either a gynaecology or endocrinology clinic and should be closely monitored by your GP.

It is imperative that women with POI get access to the most up-to-date treatment and appropriate psychological support. We need to continue to advocate to improve resources for women with POI, especially when it comes to accessing proper medical care, psychological support and funded assisted reproductive technology for fertility treatment.

Fertility

One of the hardest parts of a POI diagnosis is the impact on fertility. While 5 per cent of women diagnosed with POI may still fall pregnant, it can be very challenging and distressing. Many other routes are available today, like donor eggs and surrogacy. So do your homework here and don't just think about what your country of residence offers. Please see Resources for more on POI.

Induced menopause

After breast cancer in 2013, I had to go on tamoxifen after treatment and was told I would go into pre-menopause straight away – that was all I was told. It was hard, as I didn't know what my body was going through and had no one to help support my journey. During this time, I experienced very bad hot flushes, night sweats, brain fog, palpitations, aches and pains, low libido, anger, sadness, and at times felt I was going mad as I had so much rage against my partner. It was very difficult.

I was told 'no' to HRT by my surgeon.

I fought so hard to get vaginal oestrogen from my new GP, but she just kept treating each symptom rather than look at it as menopause-related.

I spoke to my consultant during check-ups and mentioned brain fog. I was told, 'Yes, we hear this from a lot of women – we can put you on an antidepressant.' I told them I wasn't depressed, just staring into space a lot and had no motivation.

I spoke to my GP about other symptoms and was told, 'Google may help.' I felt powerless, so I decided to do my own research, and I am still learning to this day about being in menopause.

– Marianne

Whether it's due to surgery or medical treatment, induced menopause is a far more challenging experience for most compared to natural menopause. Unfortunately, little thought or preparation is given to women undergoing these treatments, and they are often left in the dark as to what happens after the procedure or treatment.

Surgical menopause may result in symptoms coming on very quickly, whereas medical menopause can happen over a time frame of weeks or months. I would urge any woman facing the decision to have surgery to sit down with your consultant and discuss fully what the surgery entails and what the options are.

Also, remember that you are more than your organs. So many women say they feel sadness at the loss of their uterus, a loss of their femininity. But it is an organ: it does not define who you are.

Surgical menopause

Surgical menopause catapults you into cliff-edge menopause and you may bypass perimenopause altogether (unless you're already in it). It is fast, it is challenging and it is scary.

It spirals into a more intense menopause and is also associated with an increased risk of cardiovascular disease, osteoporosis and dementia, particularly when it occurs before the age of forty-five (the average age of perimenopause).

Bilateral oophorectomy: This is when the ovaries are removed, causing surgical menopause. This surgery is becoming more common due to progress in genetic testing to identify the BRCA gene. BRCA carriers are at a high risk of breast and/or ovarian cancer. If you are having a hysterectomy (see below) and are post-menopause then it is likely your ovaries will also be removed. This will eliminate your risk of ovarian cancer and, as you are post-menopause, may not impact your symptoms.

Total hysterectomy and bilateral salpingo-oophorectomy: In this surgery, the uterus, cervix, ovaries and fallopian tubes are removed, triggering menopause. Other surgeries, such as hysterectomy and ovarian cyst removal, while not directly causing menopause, can have an impact and may result in menopause happening early.

Hysterectomy: Removal of the uterus can also have an impact on blood flow to the ovaries and there may be local inflammation as tissues heal. In the past, the general practice was to remove the ovaries when a hysterectomy was being performed. If your surgeon advises removal of the ovaries (oophorectomy), it is important to understand why. If they are removed pre-menopause then you lose the hormone production your ovaries would be supplying – your natural hormones are gone. The preference would be to allow your body to produce these essential hormones naturally for as long as possible. If you are post-menopause, removal of the ovaries won't have the same impact, as your ovaries are no longer working optimally. This will also protect you from the risk of ovarian cancer. It's a matter of weighing up what stage you are at and the risks versus the benefits, taking guidance from your surgeon. In the case of a hysterectomy with no oophorectomy, also known as a partial hysterectomy, if you notice a rhythm to your menopause symptoms – for example, if headaches come on at the same time each month – you could still be going through a menstrual cycle without an actual period. If your ovaries are still in place, this can happen.

Ovarian-cyst removal: This surgery can also result in some of a normal ovary and the follicles it is storing being removed, which may impact blood flow to the ovaries.

Before any of the above surgeries, ensure you discuss the aftermath with your consultant and understand your options. For those who are able to use HRT safely, a discussion should be had prior to surgery so you are aware of the next steps. Ideally, you would receive counselling and support prior to and after surgery so that you are informed of the impact on your hormones, what to expect and what your treatment options are.

Medical menopause

Medical or chemical menopause occurs when medications impact your oestrogen production.

Radiation or chemotherapy: These treatments can also trigger menopause over a period of weeks. This can be a temporary or permanent menopause and will depend on how close you are to actual menopause itself.

Tamoxifen: This is commonly used for a person with oestrogen positive breast cancer, as it inhibits the growth of oestrogen. Any sign of abnormal bleeding when on tamoxifen must be investigated, as it can act like oestrogen on the uterus.

GnRH agonists: These are medications that keep the ovaries from making oestrogen and progesterone. They stop ovulation and production of these hormones. They are commonly used for endometriosis, breast cancer, fibroids and uterine tumours. If given for fibroids or endometriosis you may still, under the supervision of your consultant, be able to use small doses of oestrogen. Common forms are Zoladex and Leuprolide.

Aromatase inhibitors: These are used for oestrogen positive breast cancer and basically stop all production of oestrogen throughout your body – in the ovaries and also the adrenal glands. Aches and pains throughout the body are very common with this medication. Magnesium may be of benefit to counteract this.

EARLY MENOPAUSE IN THE WORKPLACE

Betty (53) to Clare (32): 'I'm suffering so badly today – I'm exhausted, as I got no sleep last night. I am so tired of night sweats. Oh, but sure you wouldn't know anything about that – you're a young one'

Clare (diagnosed with POI at 21): 'Actually, I do. I get night sweats nearly every night and I get brain fog daily.'

I find it really hard at work that no one understands what I am going through. Older colleagues think I am joking when I tell them I am in menopause and younger friends are talking about babies. It's very hard. It took me a long time to open up to Betty.

– Clare

Menopause can impact all ages: it is imperative that this is understood in all workplaces. Conversations like the above can be very distressing to women with early menopause in any form.

Your symptoms of menopause will most likely impact your work life, and you will need support. However, depending on your employer, you may feel reluctant to inform them of your diagnosis. You need time to let it settle with you first, so you can get a handle on how your body is adapting to this change and, most importantly, how you are feeling emotionally. Disclosing your early menopause is your call – only do it when and if you feel ready. Whether or not to inform your employer is a personal choice, but at a minimum, it would be great to have the support of one or two work colleagues who understand what you are experiencing.

Thankfully, workplaces, especially in Ireland and the UK, are opening up this conversation, knowing that it is important to support women going through all forms of menopause. However, we still have a long road to go to ensure support in all work environments.

If you do decide to inform your employer, you should provide them with some resources so they can understand. This is a great opportunity to familiarise yourself with your health insurance policy, your employee assistance programme (EAP) and any additional support you can avail of through these years. (See Chapter 13 for more.)

* * *

Having spoken with thousands of people across multiple countries, I firmly believe natural menopause is a privilege, as the earlier forms of menopause come with additional challenges. However, much help is now available, and there are several ways you can support yourself through your early menopause. Throughout the remainder of this book, unless stated otherwise, any practical suggestions and options can be applied to early menopause also.

Part 2: Diving In

3

Symptoms – an overview

'I feel like a bus has run over me.' 'I don't know who I am any more'. 'I just feel off-kilter and not myself.' These are just some of the things I hear from women in relation to their menopause experience. The symptoms of menopause can make you feel lost at sea, facing dark troubled waters, at least until you get a handle on what is happening, until you can understand the hormonal havoc that may be blasting its way through your body. Or maybe you are one of the lucky 25 per cent of women who go through menopause with no symptoms, or symptoms so mild you barely notice them!

Perimenopause is often slow and gradual, so it can take you unawares, and only in hindsight will you see the red flags that were waving. Understanding perimenopause is the key to unlocking this complex mystery and the symptoms that may present.

If you google the symptoms of menopause you will see anywhere upwards of thirty-six – my current list contains over fifty. My advice is to think of symptoms as clouds. They are not constant, but passing through. They can be fleeting or they can stay awhile longer, but eventually 'this too shall pass'.

It's now widely accepted that no two women will have the same experience of menopause. Every story is different, and each journey and symptom experienced is personal and not always easy to talk about. Who wants to discuss loss of confidence, a lack of interest in the bedroom, dryness everywhere and those awful mood swings? It's hard.

SYMPTOMS OF MENOPAUSE
PSYCHOLOGICAL (CHAPTER 12)
Anxiety
Low mood
Depression
Mood swings
Irritability
Crying spells
Loss of confidence
Reduced self-esteem
Loss of zest, joy for life
Panic Attacks
Sleep issues (Chapter 4)
Loss of libido (Chapter 6)
BRAIN FUNCTION (CHAPTER 8)
Brain fog
Memory loss
Concentration issues
VASOMOTOR SYMPTOMS (CHAPTER 9)
Hot flushes
Night sweats
Cold flushes
GENITOURINARY (CHAPTER 5)
Vaginal/vulval dryness, soreness, inflammation (burning sensation)
Skin thinning or splitting
Labia shrinking
Clitoral shrinking/pain
Painful smear test
Watery discharge
Abnormal vaginal bleeding

Painful sex
Bleeding after sex
Painful episiotomy scar
Recurring UTIs
Urge incontinence
Stress incontinence
Passing urine more often during the day and at night
Pelvic organ prolapse
GENERAL PHYSICAL SYMPTOMS
Changing periods
Weight gain (Chapter 10)
Tiredness
Migraines
Palpitations (Chapter 11)
Aching joints (Chapter 7)
Restless leg syndrome (Chapter 7)
Digestive issues (Chapter 19)
Histamine intolerance – increased allergies
Electric shock
Dizziness
Dry eyes/burning mouth syndrome
Dry mouth
Tinnitus
Thinning hair
Dry, itchy skin
Changing body odour
Frozen shoulder

The great news is that there is much you can do to support yourself through these years.

Many of the symptoms listed above have their own dedicated chapters, and we will cover the rest in the following pages.

> I have endured an array of other common symptoms but it always irritates me when the GP and media trot out night sweats and brain fog as if that's the only thing that women get.
>
> – Anonymous

CHANGING PERIODS

'My periods are still regular so I can't be in menopause' – let's bust this myth, fast. You can be in perimenopause even if your cycles have not yet changed, or have changed so slightly that you don't notice. As you progress through perimenopause, your periods will change in flow and become more irregular.

What to expect in the early years

Your periods may change by just a few days in the early years, until they start to go 'missing' for a few weeks or months. A healthy period should follow a cycle length of anything from twenty-one to thirty-five days. You will know what your normal length is, and using an app to track your periods can be helpful at this time. Over time, the duration between periods will be longer and the flow will also change – it can become heavier for a while before being lighter too. In summary, it's unpredictable.

What is a normal flow?

It's hard to measure! The average period is around 50ml and lasts three to seven days, with five being the ideal. Each sanitary pad or tampon holds about 5ml of blood, so ten pads or tampons. A heavy period is over 80ml.

When is a period too heavy?

You will be familiar with your regular flow and what is normal for you. When you are replacing your tampons or sanitary pads more often than before, that's an indication your period is getting heavier. It is worth keeping an eye on this, as it can impact your life in many ways – worry around having accidents could result in increased social anxiety, not to mention the impact it may have on your iron levels.

'Flooding' is used to describe heavy bleeding (hypermenorrhoea or menorrhagia) that occurs in a relatively short space of time – 25 per cent of women report having experienced heavy periods during menopause. Heavy cycles can also be due to other causes that require specific treatment, like fibroids, endometrial polyps and thyroid issues.

There are some red flags with bleeding. Watch out for:

- Having to replace a tampon or pad within the hour and heavy bleeding lasting over four hours
- The appearance of large clots
- Bleeding going on for over two weeks
- Feeling dizzy, breathless or exhausted
- Spotting/bleeding after sex

For any of the above, please consult your GP. Any sign of bleeding in the post-menopause years should be investigated.

Acupuncture and herbs can be investigated for this symptom. The Mirena coil is often prescribed for heavy bleeding also. If you experience heavy periods, investigate taking an iron supplement.

TIREDNESS

You think you'll just take a few minutes to sit down and have a breather … soon enough the eyes droop and you are fast asleep – and you're only halfway through the day. The exhaustion you might feel in these years can be from a combination of symptoms: loss of sleep, changing hormones, how you are actually feeling – it is hard to feel energised when your mood is low – not to mention other symptoms like aches and pains, headaches, brain fog, recurring colds and sleep. Many of these symptoms can also be a signpost for chronic fatigue syndrome.

You want to understand what is causing the tiredness – after all, we can't blame menopause or our age for everything. Try to rule out low iron, thyroid issues and B12 deficiency, as these are all big hitters when it comes to exhaustion. A blood test can get to the bottom of these.

Low iron/anaemia

Our blood is key in menopause – we want to be making good blood every day. It's what fuels our bodies. Many symptoms of low iron look similar to perimenopause – exhaustion, brain fog, weight gain, anxiety, palpitations and cycle issues.

Thyroid issues

Thyroid imbalance is common in women and, again, many of the symptoms are very similar to menopause – anxiety, panic attacks, palpitations, constipation, dryness, weight changes (up or down) and tiredness, to name just a few. The thyroid gland can become unbalanced in these years and can go low (hypothyroid) or high (hyperthyroid). In menopause, it starts to work even harder to keep your body on an even keel. A key distinguishing factor with a thyroid imbalance in menopause is the feeling of cold. If your thyroid is out of balance, your doctor will work with you to find the right levels of the required medication.

You can also support your thyroid health by following a good diet and taking regular exercise. Selenium and zinc are key for optimum thyroid health.

Vitamin B12

This is an essential ingredient in making healthy blood, a deficiency of which will result in extreme tiredness. You may not get enough in your diet, certain medications (notably, some antibiotics and anti-seizure medications) may interfere with its absorption, and digestive issues may impact it.

The first step is to ensure you are getting enough through your food – fish, eggs, meat, poultry, dairy and fortified foods are good sources. If you are vegetarian or vegan, you need to pay extra attention to your levels of B12. Also if you drink alcohol in excess, you need to be mindful, as alcohol impacts the absorption of B12 into the body.

Is it burnout?

You're feeling exhausted, sleep is an issue, your concentration is impacted, and you have headaches and a loss of zest. That sounds pretty perimenopausal, doesn't it? But these are also symptoms of burnout. This is one of the reasons I would encourage you to look at stress in your life (see Chapter 12) and take steps to address this first and foremost. Once you start to see things more clearly, you will be in a much better position to judge perimenopause versus burnout.

MIGRAINES

Migraines are those headaches that leave you in pieces, shattered and exhausted beyond belief. Experience of migraines can differ from one person to the next, and they can become heightened in perimenopause and taper off in the post-menopausal period. Women are three times more likely to get migraines than men.

How do I know if I have a migraine?

Migraines are a type of headache with a neurological basis and can be extremely debilitating. Often people will describe an 'aura' that precedes or comes with a migraine. It is much more than a bad headache – it is generally characterised by severe one-sided pain, in addition to nausea and/ or vomiting and vision changes. Generally, there is a great sensitivity to light and sound, and sometimes the sensory issues can extend to smell and touch. Migraines can be episodic – that is, they come on without warning and their frequency is random and variable, lasting anywhere from a few hours to three days, or longer in some cases. Chronic migraines mean you get more than fifteen headaches in any given month and eight of these would be classic migraines.

Practical steps

CoQ10: It is currently understood that migraines involve two factors – oversensitivity of the brain to normal stimuli and an inflammatory response within the brain. Calcitonin gene-related peptide (CGRP) is released when the sensory nerve endings in the nerves and blood vessels are stimulated. This causes the blood vessels to dilate, including those in the pain-sensitive outer membrane covering the brain. CoQ10 (Coenzyme Q10) works by lowering this peptide. Human studies have shown that CoQ10 at doses of 150–300mg daily can help migraine sufferers by preventing occurrence, reducing the duration of a migraine by 50 per cent and reducing the monthly frequency – it also tends to be effective without side effects. The form called 'ubiquinol' enables higher levels of CoQ10 to enter the bloodstream. In 2015, the Canadian Headache Society listed CoQ10 as a recommendation for migraines, along with B2 and magnesium. The Migraine Association of Ireland also lists these three supplements as being helpful for migraines.

B2 (riboflavin) plays a big role in the work of the mitochondria – the energy powerhouses of the cells. These act like a digestive system within the cells, taking in nutrients and breaking them down, creating energy for the cells. An imbalance in the mitochondria is thought to play a part in the occurrence of migraines. Sources of riboflavin include organ meats and other meat, certain dairy products, green leafy veggies, beans and legumes, and nuts and seeds.

Magnesium has been widely shown to help with migraines. Like B2, it plays a key role in mitochondrial energy production. It is also key in muscle relaxation, enhancing communication between cells, and serotonin and other neurotransmitter production and regulation. While magnesium used to be abundant in our food chain, through the soil, this is no longer the case. In addition, today's diets tend to include increased amounts of sugar, fat and processed foods, all of which affect the absorption of magnesium into our bodies. (See Chapter 16 for more.)

HRT can have a role to play, with some caveats. As HRT is generally very effective for hot flushes and night sweats, which are often triggers for migraines, helping these symptoms can indirectly prevent migraines. But some types of HRT may actually cause migraines. This generally happens with the oral forms, so transdermal forms would be a better option if you are already experiencing migraines. The transdermal patch offers a steady supply, which works well for many migraine sufferers.

Look for triggers: Keep a diary of when migraines come on and note what you ate beforehand and anything else that was happening. Note the duration and severity also.

Food: Chemicals contained in many foods today can be a trigger for migraines – for example, tyramine (in cheese), phenylethylamine (in chocolate), tyrosine, MSG, aspartame, caffeine, sulphites, nitrates and histamine (in wine and beer).

Look at your lifestyle: Ongoing chronic stress can be a key factor in migraines. Make the lifestyle adjustments you need and then monitor to see if they help. For example, if lack of sleep might be a trigger, then note what happens when good sleep hygiene is introduced.

Relaxation techniques can be very helpful, as can cognitive behavioural therapy (CBT).

Essential oils: Rosemary and lavender mixed together with a carrier oil and rubbed onto the neck and temples can help. You could also add a drop of each to a tissue and inhale when needed.

Exercise: Many migraine sufferers benefit from a daily exercise schedule.

Acupuncture can improve migraine for many people.

Eyewear: If you are experiencing migraine, consider amber eyeglasses, which help with the blue light emitted from computer screens.

Medication: Speak with your GP, who will advise on medications that may support you.

If you experience severe pain, paralysis down one side of the body or face, speech difficulties, double vision or a rash, make sure to contact your doctor to rule out a more serious underlying condition.

ELECTRIC SHOCK

It's like a sudden jolt, a blast of electricity through your body. For the majority of women it just comes and goes, but sometimes it may signal that a hot flush is on the way.

There has been little research in this area, and these electric shocks may be a combination of ageing and hormonal changes. Key here would be oestrogen: as hormones go out of kilter, messages to the brain can be impacted or short-circuited, resulting in a sensation similar to an electric shock or tingling throughout the body. Low levels of B12 can also cause this.

And like many symptoms, it may not be due to menopause – if you are feeling it down your leg, it could be related to a disc that is herniated. Osteoporosis in your spine can increase your risk of this symptom, so that's another good reason to get a DXA scan and check your bone health (see Chapter 7).

DIZZINESS

Vertigo/dizziness/benign paroxysmal positional vertigo (BBPV) happens when your head position changes, causing short dizzy spells. To understand this more we need to look at otoconia. These are bio-crystals that live in your inner ear. They interact with the small sensory hair cells that line the inner ear. BBPV happens when these are out of balance. This can happen due to low oestrogen, low calcium and a loss of these sensory hair cells, which happens with ageing.

In a study of 935 women in Nebraska, 50 per cent reported experiencing vertigo (dizziness) and impacts on balance after menopause. In addition, 32 per cent of women who had a hysterectomy and 22 per cent of women who had their ovaries removed also reported an increase in this symptom.

The study concluded that when hormone levels change, this can result in a change to the bio-crystals and they move to another part of the ear (the semicircular canals). When they move into the canals, they send incorrect signals to your brain about how you are positioned, giving you that spinning sensation so typical of vertigo.

While dizziness is not one of the most common symptoms of menopause, if you do experience it, you will know how it can impact your life. It's not just feeling dizzy: it can also cause nausea and vomiting and affect your balance, with the greatest risk being that you may fall and cause yourself an injury.

Some steps to take:

- Visit an osteopath – this can be a great help with vertigo.
- Investigate the Epley manoeuvre – a series of movements designed to dislodge the bio-crystals from the semicircular canals.
- Incorporate balance exercises such as tai chi, Pilates or yoga into your weekly routine.
- Look at your calcium and magnesium intake: magnesium helps to expand blood vessels – with menopause they can become more constricted.
- Walk barefoot! Your feet also play a role in balance, and walking barefoot will improve the proprioceptive neural input to the brain from receptors in your muscles and joints, which will lead to a better awareness of your body's position in space and may even reduce pain.

It's also good to keep all the joints and muscles working as they should to maintain strength, stability and range of movement in the foot and ankle.

DRY EYES

There is nothing equal to the dryness of menopause. Dry eyes are caused by problems with your tears. We all have a tear film that covers and lubricates our eyes. This film is made up of water, oil and mucus. When you don't produce enough tears, this can result in a dry, gritty, irritated feeling in your eye. It can be accompanied by a stinging, burning, hot sensation and blurred vision. As we get older, tear production naturally declines, and women post-menopause are very susceptible to this symptom. More research is required into this area but current thinking points to a decline in both androgens (the hormones both men and women have) and oestrogen having an impact here.

Several triggers may be creating dry eyes. The common causes are a reduction in actual tear production, tears drying up (dry air, contact lenses or allergies can cause this) or poor-quality tears.

What can you do?

HRT: There's no clear answer for this, with some studies showing that long-term HRT actually increases the risk and severity of dry-eye symptoms.

Omega-7 has a great affinity with mucous membranes and may help here. See Chapter 5 for more.

Speak to your pharmacist: Some over-the-counter medications are available to treat chronic dry-eye problems. In most cases, artificial tears will be enough to ease your symptoms. Just watch out for drops with preservatives, as these can irritate your eyes if you use them too much. Eye drops that reduce redness can also be irritating if used too often. Eye drops without preservatives are safe to use more than four times per day.

Talk to your doctor: There may be prescription medications that can help.

Remember, eyes are a key part of our long-term health, so looking after them is all-important. Try these practical steps:

- Limit your screen time – if you work at a computer all day, remember to take breaks. Close your eyes for a few minutes or blink repeatedly for a few seconds.
- Protect your eyes – wear sunglasses and a hat when outside. Sunglasses that wrap around the face can block wind and dry air. They can help when you're exercising too.
- Avoid triggers – irritants like smoke and pollen can make your symptoms more severe.
- Use a humidifier – keeping the air in your home or office moist may help.
- Eat right – a good diet rich in omega-3 fatty acids and vitamin A can encourage healthy tear production.
- Avoid contact lenses (if possible) as they can make dry eyes worse.
- Exercise your eyes – for general eye health, get into a habit of doing a mix of these daily eye exercises:
  - » Close – Pause – Open – Relax: first, gently close your eyes, keep them closed for two seconds, then open slowly and relax them. Repeat this five times.
  - » Follow this with Close – Pause – Squeeze – Open – Relax: gently close your eyes, pause for two seconds, squeeze tightly for two seconds, then open and relax. Repeat this five times.

Your vision and spatial awareness may also change. This can result in bumping into things more often and parking a car becoming more of a challenge; driving can become more stressful due to the changes in how we perceive other cars. Your vision may be being impacted by fluctuating oestrogen levels, so that's a good reason to get your eyes tested.

DRY MOUTH

It may not be just before you speak to a large audience or when you're feeling nervous: in menopause, dry mouth can happen at any time, and many do not see this as a symptom of menopause. The official term, xerostomia, means a reduction in saliva produced in the mouth and a sensation of dryness. Saliva is an important part of immune health: it protects your mouth against harmful bacteria, so producing the right amount is crucial. When production is impacted, you are open to tooth decay, gum inflammation, cavities and infections. A dry mouth will also impact your sense of taste and can make your mouth feel sore. It can extend to your throat and lips, making you feel thirsty constantly and sometimes even hoarse. (Burning mouth syndrome is related to this too – see below.)

Why does it happen?

Oestrogen and saliva production are linked, so the decline in oestrogen may impact saliva production for some women. Stress and ongoing anxiety will also trigger this symptom. Steps to take include:

- Making dental hygiene a must and paying frequent visits to your dentist.
- Staying hydrated.
- Keeping your lips moist – dry mouth will cause dry lips.
- Chewing gum – this will help produce more saliva in the mouth.
- Being aware of foods that may make it worse – they will vary from person to person.
- Monitoring your caffeine and alcohol intake – both will dry your mouth out further.
- Quitting smoking – smoking slows down your production of saliva and has an overall negative impact on your health.
- Looking for other triggers – medication you are taking, anxiety levels, dehydration or other medical conditions that may cause this symptom (for example, Sjogren's syndrome).

BURNING MOUTH SYNDROME

Worst was the burning mouth and blood blisters in the mouth, and the other is the terror of driving on a motorway because there is something there related to anxiety or changes in spatial awareness that can catch you and cause extreme distress when driving.

– Anon

Not a common symptom, but bothersome if you have it, burning mouth syndrome is a sensation of burning or scalding in the mouth that can be felt in your gums, tongue, lips, the inside of your cheeks or the roof of your mouth. It can impact your sense of taste and can also be accompanied by a dry mouth. Again, don't just blame menopause! It can be a sign of other conditions such as allergies, diabetes or thyroid, side effects of medication or nutritional deficiencies, especially of B vitamins. Incorporating the steps outlined for dry mouth may help.

TINNITUS

I had bad tinnitus. I was giving out about the neighbours leaving on extractor fans until I realised when I stayed in another house that the noise was still there. I had bad rashes – I was on antihistamines every day and using an anti-itch cream. I was working my way through an exclusion diet to see what I was allergic to. I had funny tastes in my mouth and gum recession despite different kinds of toothpaste and mouthwashes.

– Roisín

Hearing changes come with age, but they can be accelerated in menopause, and hearing is important for long-term health. (For more on this in relation to the impact on brain health and cognitive function, see Chapter 8.)

Tinnitus is characterised by a hissing, ringing noise – sounds that are not actually happening externally. It can be caused by damage to the inner ear or it may happen as a result of the hormonal changes in menopause. We have oestrogen receptors in our ear cells and auditory pathways, but it is still unclear how oestrogen impacts hearing – research is ongoing. Since both generally happen at the same time and age, it makes it harder to know if one causes the other or if both are factors.

There are limited studies in this area, but some suggest that HRT can actually worsen the symptoms of tinnitus. A 2017 research paper published in the North American Menopause Society's journal claims HRT is associated with a higher risk of hearing loss. Researchers analysed 80,972 women and found that the use of oral HRT for women who go through menopause at a later age than average also had greater hearing loss. As with everything related to HRT, it is crucial to make an informed decision and discuss the risks and benefits with your GP.

Try these practical steps to help with tinnitus:

- Practice good ear hygiene (see Chapter 8).
- Look for any triggers – what makes it worse or kicks it off? Keeping a menopause journal is really handy here.
- Check any medication you are taking and look for side effects of hearing changes – some painkillers, antibiotics and antidepressants can make this worse.
- Introduce white noise – if the tinnitus is bothering you, the calming sounds of nature, waves and rain can be a welcome distraction.
- Relaxation can also help – try any of the forms discussed throughout this book.

SKIN CHANGES

Oestrogen plays a key role in the health and appearance of your skin and is responsible for many of the things that we associate with youthfulness – think firm, smooth, supple skin with that enviable radiance. As we go through menopause and our oestrogen levels decline, this has a profound impact on our skin health. It is also estimated that in the first five years of menopause we lose 30 per cent of our skin's collagen, the all-important protein that gives skin structure and support. This loss leads to wrinkled, slightly sagging and more sensitive skin, partly because of this thinning.

The decline in oestrogen also brings about a decline in our own natural hydrating agents, like sebum, hyaluronic acid and ceramides, which translates physically into that feeling of dryness and tightness. This is not just confined to the face – skin on the body can also feel a lot drier and tighter. Testosterone can start to become relatively stronger in the body because of the female hormones dropping, which can lead to acne and excess hair on the cheeks, neck and chin.

Formication is intense itching of the skin, as though insects are crawling on it. It is not a common symptom but it can happen. It can also be a symptom of diabetes or shingles and a side effect of stopping some medications like antidepressants.

Understanding what happens around the menopause and how that impacts your skin health is key to understanding what we actually have to do to address the skin changes you might be experiencing. Far from popular belief, it is not game over when it comes to the appearance of your complexion. Now is the time to reassess your skincare regime to ensure it's working to meet your needs and concerns, with the emphasis on being gentle – you don't want to dry out skin even more or compromise the delicate skin barrier. Look for collagen-stimulating skincare ingredients like vitamin C, peptides and retinoids, and ensure you adopt the daily habit of applying a broad-spectrum sunscreen to protect your skin from accelerated ageing. If you need guidance, please seek the advice of a skincare specialist who will be able to advise and recommend what is best suited for you and your skin.

– Sherna Malone, skin health specialist and facialist

HAIR CHANGES

Hair loss, thinning and growing in places you don't want are all very common. Generally, hair loss and thinning happen around the front of the head, but it can be all over. And then, of course, the famous chin and facial hairs may start to appear.

Our hair is always falling out – that is the cycle it goes through: new hair grows, hangs around for a while (resting stage) and then falls out. It needs oestrogen to help with this growth cycle. Other underlying conditions can also impact hair so remember to check for iron, thyroid and chronic stress. Look at your nutritional intake and up your protein and iron (leafy green vegetables, beetroot, pumpkin seeds, chickpeas, whole lentils, flaxseeds), invest in a good shampoo and conditioner, and use a hair mask weekly (homemade or shop bought): all will support your hair. If you colour your hair, look for ammonia-free colour that will be easier on your scalp. Be mindful of the impact of heating tools, like straighteners, on your hair too. The key vitamins for healthy hair are B vitamins, biotin, vitamin C and zinc.

NAILS

Our nails are made of a protein called keratin. Nails are strong and evenly formed when the body is in good health. Your keratin production is out of balance if your nails are showing signs of brittleness. Declining oestrogen also makes your nails more dehydrated, which may lead to weaker, brittle, dry nails. Many women show me ridges in their nails that have developed with age and are now more noticeable.

To keep your nails healthy through these years, use a good moisturiser throughout the day – carry a tube in your bag – and use an intensive hand moisturiser last thing at night (almond oil is lovely here). If you are doing housework, make sure to wear gloves, as they will protect you from harsh chemicals. A healthy diet will also benefit your nails, especially foods rich in omega-3, zinc and biotin.

If you are a fan of shellac nail polish, remember to not leave it on too long, as it is not nourishing your nails. When you are having it applied, put an SPF cream on your hands to protect you from the damage of the lamps. UV or LED lamps emit UVA rays that have been linked to an increased risk of skin cancer.

CHANGING BODY ODOUR

No, it's not your perfume that has changed, it's the changes coursing through your body. Up until perimenopause, I could easily have gone days without wearing deodorant – I rarely perspired unless I was exercising. Perimenopause changed all that. It can feel like your perspiration smells stronger, and you notice it like you never did before.

When we delve into hot flushes, you will see all about thermoregulation (see Chapter 9). This zone is reduced in menopause, which means your body sweats more at lower temperatures. As anxiety has a large part to play in these years, it can also add fuel to the fire. For some women, as the hormones change, it can be that at certain stages you have more testosterone going through your body, and this can make your body odour smell stronger. This is unavoidable so all you can do is be prepared – keep deodorants in easy reach!

When choosing a deodorant, aim for naturally derived ingredients – as you're using this regularly, it is good to be mindful of what is going into your body.

FROZEN SHOULDER

Another symptom that I've had on the menopause journey has been a frozen left shoulder which was absolutely debilitating. It took a full year from start to finish and shook me to the core. My doctor definitively refused to make any link to menopause but the female physio I attended was in no doubt. There are a high number of ladies in my age range who have suffered frozen shoulders, so I find it amazing that doctors can't see the link.

– Anonymous

Frozen shoulder happens when the tissue around your shoulder joint becomes inflamed, causing it to become tight and triggering pain. The joint has a liquid called synovial fluid, like the oil in a car, helping it to move smoothly. If the joint is damaged it may lose some of this fluid and movement becomes limited, giving rise to the name 'frozen'. There is no confirmation of a direct link with menopause, but as oestrogen affects joint health it may contribute to this issue.

HISTAMINE INTOLERANCE – INCREASED ALLERGIES

While we can't blame menopause for everything, hormonal changes do affect the production of histamine. This can impact how your skin feels and cause food sensitivity, alcohol sensitivity, asthma or runny nose and eyes. You can wake up one morning after a glass of red wine the night before, sneezing to beat the band or with a tissue permanently in hand as your nose constantly drips.

Histamine is a chemical that exists in cells in your body called mast cells. It is an integral part of your immune system. When your body is allergic to a particular substance, such as food or dust, the immune system mistakenly believes that this usually harmless substance is actually a threat to the body. In an attempt to protect the body, the immune system starts a chain reaction that prompts the mast cells to release histamine and other chemicals into the bloodstream. The histamine then acts on a person's eyes, nose, throat, lungs, skin or gastrointestinal tract, causing allergy symptoms by making the blood vessels expand and the area to become inflamed (internally or externally). The most common symptoms are sneezing or wheezing, as mucous builds up in the airways. This response by your body is known as histamine intolerance.

But it has impacts aside from the typical allergic reaction. It can cause heavy periods and period pain because histamine triggers more oestrogen to be produced, and then the mast cells in the uterus release two chemicals, called prostaglandins and heparin, both of which can cause heavy periods. It's a feedback loop between oestrogen and histamine, with oestrogen stimulating histamine, and histamine telling the ovaries to create more oestrogen, and the cycle continues.

What you will notice is that many of these symptoms mirror those of perimenopause, so it's a matter of determining which is causing them. The key symptoms include insomnia, headaches, migraines, PMT, mood swings, heavy periods, painful periods, breast tenderness, anxiety, hives, itchy skin and urinary issues. Watch out too for when you notice the symptoms more – if you are still having cycles it can be traced back to your oestrogen and progesterone. Remember how these two balance each other – as progesterone drops, oestrogen becomes higher. This also explains why you may feel the side effects of histamine more at different stages of the menopause transition.

There are a few practical steps you can take to reduce histamine:

- Avoid foods high in histamine – fermented foods, such as kimchi and sauerkraut, some mature cheeses, aged meats and alcohol are very high.
- Increase your intake of brassica vegetables – these will support liver detoxification of oestrogen (where there is excess oestrogen). Go for broccoli, cauliflower, kale, cabbage and brussels sprouts.
- Avoid inflammatory foods – these take an added toll on your immune system and can trigger a further release of histamine. Foods to watch here are gluten, sugar, fried foods, processed foods, red meat and dairy.
- Look at what foods might trigger a reaction for you. Pineapples, bananas and strawberries are common culprits.
- Increase your intake of antihistamine foods – many of these contain what we call prebiotics (good bacteria). Go for onions and garlic (if allowed), turmeric, ginger, peppermint, thyme, oregano, watercress, pomegranate, basil, carrots, broccoli, fennel and chamomile.
- Know your food source – foods high in preservatives, additives and/or chemical sprays may have an impact.
- Look after your gut health – gut dysbiosis and small intestine bacterial

overgrowth (SIBO) can trigger histamine. These are conditions caused by an overgrowth of harmful bacteria in the gut and small intestine and can lower your tolerance to histamine.

- Be kind to your liver! It does a great amount of work for you every day and we should give it more support (see Chapter 19 for ways to do this).
- Try antihistamine medications – these help to fight symptoms caused by the release of histamine during an allergic reaction.
- Manage stress – this may increase the levels of histamine in your body.
- Stay hydrated.
- Consult a dietitian or nutritional therapist: they may help identify your trigger foods.

IS IT FIBROMYALGIA OR MENOPAUSE?

Fibromyalgia is an illness that causes pain throughout the body. It can result in sleep problems, fatigue and emotional and mental difficulties – symptoms that may overlap with those of menopause. But the pain of fibromyalgia is what sets it apart. Working with a doctor or consultant experienced in this area is key. Studies are ongoing in relation to fibromyalgia, but for now, the main areas to look at in relieving and helping the symptoms are as follows:

- Reduce stress as much as possible.
- Support your gut – feed it well, especially with prebiotics and probiotics.
- Protein is often lacking in the diet of fibromyalgia patients, and it is especially important to consume this early in the morning, so look at your breakfast and ensure you incorporate protein at the start of your day. Protein is not just for building muscles: it is essential for the immune system and helps keep blood sugar levels balanced (they can go haywire in perimenopause).
- CoQ10 is a key component of energy production. It is very hard to get through diet so a supplement is the best way to go.
- Glucose and fat are needed by cell mitochondria to produce energy.

Getting the fat into the mitochondria is not a simple process – it might need a little assistance to carry it along the way. That helper is acetyl-L-carnitine, which can be very helpful to fibromyalgia sufferers and is found in red meat, poultry, fish and milk.

- Magnesium can help with muscle stiffness and also helps energy production in the body (see Chapter 16).
- Antioxidants will support the all-important mitochondria.
- If gas and bloating are symptoms, peppermint oil may be helpful. Ensure it is enteric coated – this helps it bypass the stomach, which is acidic, and get to the small intestine, which is alkaline: this is where the gas that creates the bloating is located.

ARE YOU MORE PRONE TO COLDS AND FLUS?

Our body's immune system is extremely complex. It consists of constant interactions between our glands, hormones, proteins, chemicals, white blood cells and probiotics. These all work together to protect our bodies from infections. Think of them as your personal warriors: their primary role is to ward off enemies. To perform this defensive role, the body must have good fuel and energy – this is where food, sleep, exercise, rest and the other lifestyle choices outlined in this book are essential.

In menopause, this system comes under pressure. Many different aspects of life collide to impact your immunity, making you more prone to colds, flu and allergies (as we saw with histamine changes). It's not just menopause and changing hormones: it's age, stress, sleep issues, gut health and ongoing tiredness. All of this combined with hormonal chaos leaves you susceptible to immune issues and immune disorders.

THE ROLE OF THE SYMPTOM CHECKER

With so many possible symptoms, it is a good idea to start keeping track of them and noticing what is changing in your body. I would love to see this happening from the early forties onwards, so women will be able to notice the subtle changes in these years. A symptom checker can be found in the Resources section, and now is the perfect time to grab a cup of tea and a pen and fill it out!

* * *

Now that we've covered many of the typical symptoms, let's dig a little deeper into the better-known aspects of menopause.

4

Sleep

Where do you begin when trying to get a handle on your menopause symptoms? I'm asked this question a lot, and my response is always the same: start with sleep. It is the first step to minding yourself during these years.

Deep, nourishing, restorative sleep is the foundation of thriving through menopause. Your body will perform better in the short and long term when you have good sleep habits in place. At all stages in life, restorative sleep is crucial. Our bodies love routine: they love the rhythm of it and knowing the same amount of sleep comes at the end of every day. Yes, this can be boring and, yes, we can't do it every night, but if you can aim for it most nights your body will thank you.

Sleep is vital for:

- Physical repair of the body – most of our body's soft tissue and muscle repair happens during sleep. It's a nightly immune boost for the body and an opportunity for all those good bacteria in your gut microbiome to multiply and flourish.
- Mental cognition – sleep keeps our brains sharp and focused, which helps us to learn better and enables decision-making.
- Emotional regulation and good mental health – your day is processed by your brain when you sleep.

WHAT HAPPENS WHEN WE SLEEP?

Sleep is a well-planned event. It involves several cycles (four to five 90-minute cycles is the average) of different stages each night over seven to nine hours, ideally. The stages begin with non-rapid eye movement (NREM) sleep, moving into the deep sleep stages – where deep restoration of your body happens – and finishing with a rapid eye movement (REM) sleep stage, which lasts about ten minutes initially and becomes longer throughout the night as you transition through the cycles. It is OK to have momentary awakenings during the night – this is actually normal.

The sleep–wake cycle

Three key factors come into play with the sleep–wake cycle:

- **Pressure for sleep (homeostatic drive):** Pressure builds up throughout the day, starting as soon as we wake up in the morning. The longer we are awake the stronger the pressure, and it decreases while we sleep. Think of it like an egg timer: as soon as your day starts, the sand (a chemical called adenosine) starts to fall, and by the end of the day the timer chamber is full – the pressure is maxed out. Then it will be at an all-time low after a night of good-quality restorative sleep.

- **Circadian rhythm:** Your body clock is a highly sensitive internal system that regulates a twenty-four-hour rhythm. It will make you feel awake in the morning and tired at night. This also works closely with your core body temperature, triggering it to reach its peak at about 5 p.m. and its lowest at about 5 a.m. (Temperature has a big part to play in sleep and this may be partly why it suffers so much during menopause, triggering the temperature-related issues we know as 'vasomotor' – see Chapter 9).

- **Melatonin production:** melatonin is secreted by the pineal gland and triggers your body into sleep.

We need these processes to work together to optimise sleep quality. Ideally, the number of hours you sleep should leave you feeling refreshed and alert throughout the day.

Females, the unemployed or retired, shift workers, post-menopausal women, worriers/overthinkers and those suffering from a mental health issue are more susceptible to insomnia. Unfortunately, a history of poor sleep is also related to a risk of dementia, Alzheimer's and heart disease.

> I had weeks where I would just burst into tears as I dragged myself out of bed in the morning. Sleep was gone for me. I had always loved my sleep but perimenopause just hit me like a rocket. So many days where I couldn't function – I honestly don't know how I kept my job going. It was like I was a ghost going through my life. It was the worst of all my symptoms – I'll take a hot flush any day over restless sleep.
>
> – Mary

WHY DOES SLEEP BECOME SUCH AN ISSUE IN MENOPAUSE?

Circadian rhythms are all-important when it comes to sleep, and our bodies thrive on knowing what is coming next. The unpredictability of menopause is not a favoured chapter for our bodies. Progesterone and oestrogen, as well melatonin, the other key hormone related to sleep, will impact your rhythm. Sleep disturbance can ensue and have a knock-on impact on all aspects of your life. It can start with tiredness, resulting in a rushed, or no, breakfast, thus brain fog is heightened – your memory and concentration may not be the same. If you are on the road, you may end up taking a wrong turn; at work you may lose track of what you're supposed to be doing. Add the resulting anxiety into the mix, and your confidence will be impacted too.

Sleep – understanding what is going wrong with it and how you can fix it – can be the foundation for turning your menopause symptoms around (either in tandem with the other options outlined in this book or on its own).

Key reasons you might struggle with your sleep:

- Night-time visits to the loo
- Night sweats
- Difficulty falling asleep
- Waking up wide awake during the night
- Sleep apnoea
- Depression

'A ruffled mind makes a restless pillow' – Charlotte Bronte

YOUR LIVER, STRESS AND SLEEP

Cortisol is the stress hormone that works on the liver and pancreas to maintain glucose levels. It is generally higher in the morning and lower at night. If your cortisol levels are high at night-time, it has a direct impact on your bodily functions and your sleep. The liver will be busy working when it should be doing its normal nightly tasks, and deep sleep will be elusive – simply put, your body can't relax because it's getting signals to keep it alert. We also tend to worry more at night, so a vicious cycle sets in. Understanding how you can prime your body for a deep nourishing sleep is a good place to start (see below).

Insomnia is all too common, whether in perimenopause or not, and physical or emotional symptoms are generally the reasons behind interrupted sleep. But the most common or underlying reason is stress and anxiety.

First, look at *what* is waking you up – look for the symptom and then start to dig deeper. In many cases it can be traced back to stress. (See Chapter 12 for help with this.) It's also important that sleep itself doesn't become a stressor for you – sleep is very individual and what's insufficient for one person may be plenty for another. Focus on how rested you feel.

HEALTHY SLEEP HABITS – WHERE TO START

Review your sleep habits to ensure they are conducive to sleep, but be aware that healthy habits alone may not treat a sleep problem. Many people who have excellent night-time routines in place still experience sleep issues, and it is important that establishing these habits does not add to your frustration or create added stress.

Establishing good daytime habits

Routine: Our bodies love routine. Going to bed and getting up at the same time every day gives our sleep its own routine and rhythm, which is so important, as it allows our bodies to recover from the day and gives our immune system the time to do its magic and keep us strong. Lack of sleep will increase cortisol levels, which in turn adds to your stress, so sleep is critical. Sleep regulates the immune response and lowers inflammatory cytokines. Remember, it's a twenty-four-hour cycle and a seven-day week – the weekends should be the same as the rest of the week.

Listen to your body: Go to bed when you feel tired – don't miss the time slot! Think of an overtired toddler ...

Exercise has been proven to be of great benefit for sleep. Studies have shown that exercise earlier in the morning (and outside if possible) helps to regulate the body clock and makes it easier to fall asleep early, reduces waking episodes and improves deep sleep.

Relax: Establish a relaxing night-time routine – relaxation prior to bed is essential to bring down the stress hormone, cortisol. Do some simple breathing exercises to help you drift off to sleep. For example, breathe in slowly through your nose, hold your breath for a couple of seconds, then breathe out slowly through your mouth.

Light helps get that circadian rhythm kicked off and consistent. As soon as you wake up in the morning, you want the brightest lights possible on and the curtains open wide. This sends a strong signal to your brain that it is morning and your morning rhythm is starting. At night-time, it's the converse – keep lights dim. A stroll at dusk can be of great help. Blue-light exposure from screens, lights and electronic devices will interfere with melatonin production and put your sleep out of kilter. Try to reduce screen time one to two hours before bed. These actions at either end of the day will give the body a clear sense of time and help keep your body clock in sync.

Practising good sleep habits

- A no-tech bedroom is crucial for uninterrupted sleep. Revert to a battery alarm clock.
- Keep your room cold – it does not have to be freezing: a temperature of 18–20 degrees is what you are aiming for.
- Keep your room dark.
- Don't nap during the day if you can avoid it. If you do need a nap, try to limit it to thirty minutes before 3 p.m. (unless you are on shift work, in which case, ninety-minute sleep sessions can benefit you before you head into a night shift). Napping too long or too close to bedtime reduces sleep pressure.
- No heavy meals after 8 p.m.
- Establish a social media ban from 9 p.m. Avoid looking at your phone or tablet last thing at night (see note on blue light above).
- Avoid exercising at night.
- Declutter your bedroom – it will immediately lead to a calmer mind.
- Be mindful of your caffeine and alcohol intake (see Chapter 19 for more on alcohol).

Caffeine

Philippa was suffering severe ongoing insomnia. When we met, she was doing everything right and I was puzzled as to what was causing the sleep problem, apart from the obvious possible hormonal fluctuations. After digging deeper, it emerged Philippa was pretty fond of her tea. She was, in fact, drinking twelve to fourteen cups of tea a day. This can be a common practice, but it can wreak havoc on your sleep and your anxiety and also increase hot flushes. (Note: withdrawal from a high intake of caffeine like this has to be very gradual – a cold-turkey approach is not recommended!)

Don't get me wrong – I love a cup of coffee (always decaf), but I am well aware of the problems it creates for many people. It is the enemy of sleep, making you feel alert and full of energy when all your lovely body wants to do is rest. Caffeine, if you are sensitive to it, can make you feel irritable and anxious. It is a stimulant and, like all stimulants, will increase anxiety and agitation. It is also a diuretic so will only worsen symptoms of dehydration, which are common in menopause.

Ideally, you should monitor your intake of caffeine, and if you are experiencing sleep issues I would recommend no caffeine after 1 p.m. (make that a similar distance before your bedtime if you are a shift worker). Caffeine can block the action of adenosine, a key player in sleep pressure, in your body. So while adenosine builds throughout the day and sends your body sleep signals, caffeine will confuse your body, telling it to stay alert and awake. The best time to drink caffeine is in the morning, within one hour of waking up.

Remember, too, caffeine is not just coffee – regular tea, some isotonic drinks, chocolate and some pain medications contain caffeine, and even decaffeinated coffee can still contain caffeine: it all comes down to the processing of the coffee bean and the method used. So I would urge anyone with sleep issues to first look at their caffeine intake and reduce it where needed. After 1 p.m., try a caffeine-free herbal tea – tulsi, chamomile or valerian tea can be lovely and relaxing before bed.

If you're reading this while drinking a cup of regular tea, don't feel bad! Just be aware – look for the triggers that are impacting your sleep.

NIGHT SWEATS

If you're experiencing night sweats, try some of the tips below to help:

- Have a tepid shower before bedtime and keep a glass of water beside your bed.
- A great tip from sleep expert Tom Coleman is to have a bowl of ice by the bed with a face cloth in it – if you wake up in intense heat, you can apply the cloth to your forehead, the back of your neck and your wrists.
- Wear light nightclothes made of cotton or bamboo.
- Check your bedding – often this can be making things worse. Look at the tog of the duvet – you might need a lighter one. And look at the material – cotton will be cooler than synthetic.
- Check what your mattress protector is made of if you are using one – this can be another culprit.
- Try some relaxation exercises.
- Accept the symptoms – resistance is exhausting, and you will make progress by accepting what is going on and looking for ways to relieve it.
- Discuss HRT options with your GP.

If you are experiencing the vasomotor symptoms of menopause (night sweats and hot flushes) and start a HRT regime, it is worth keeping a sleep diary so you can see if an improvement is made. Sleep issues can often still be a part of these years even when on HRT. Gabapentin and progesterone can also be investigated and taken in isolation for sleep issues in consultation with your GP.

CBT-I

Cognitive behavioural therapy specially for sleep issues is called CBT-I. This can be extremely effective for sleep problems and have a positive impact on sleep in menopause. It has been shown to be more effective compared to sleeping medication. Sleeping medication is no longer considered the first port of call when dealing with sleep issues, but it can play an important short-term role.

SLEEP AND ALZHEIMER'S

If you are familiar with the work of Dr Lisa Mosconi, you will be aware of the importance of sleep when it comes to protecting our health in the future – especially in relation to Alzheimer's and dementia. Two out of three Alzheimer's and dementia patients are women – this is something we need to be aware of. Menopause provides us with a window of opportunity to optimise our health in our later years and this is one where it takes centre stage. As we get older our sleep naturally gets lighter, and this impacts memory. But a US study showed that, in patients with amyloid build-up (a protein that accumulates in the brain), this was more than the signs of ageing, and the deep non-REM sleep was impacted. Sleep issues are now being considered a red flag for the early indicator of these illnesses.

COMMON SLEEP DISORDERS

Insomnia

This is the most common sleep disorder, affecting about 15 per cent of the population. It is classed as difficulty falling and staying asleep (which impacts your daytime activities greatly), happening three nights a week for more than three months, with no underlying medical conditions which may be causing it. Psychological triggers are common in insomnia, with the main ones being worry, anxiety and emotional distress causing a heightened fight-or-flight response that cannot calm itself when bedtime comes. Cortisol, noradrenaline and adrenaline, the fight-or-flight chemicals, all raise heart rate – excellent when you're in danger and need to escape, but not so much when you are lying in bed wanting nothing more than a calm, blissful sleep. These chemicals also trigger your metabolic rate to increase, which makes your body grow warmer, and a higher temperature is not conducive to sleep. A drop in your body's core temperature is a prerequisite to sleep starting. Knowing how to calm your mind and body down, and practising it, is a key step in your sleep routine.

There are many different sleep disorders, so if working on your sleep habits isn't helping, it is vital to get a proper diagnosis. Speaking to your GP is crucial to start you on the road to treatment.

Sleep apnoea

Sleep apnoea is a dangerous sleep disorder in which your breathing repeatedly stops and resumes while you are sleeping. If left untreated, it can lead to loud snoring, daytime fatigue and more serious issues such as heart disease or high blood pressure.

We often think of this as mostly impacting men, but after menopause it can become more common for women also. This may be due to the drop in progesterone and the increase in visceral fat that happens in menopause.

If you think you might have sleep apnoea, the key thing to look out for is snoring. If you have a partner, they might say it sounds like you're choking at different stages of the night. Other common symptoms are a dry mouth in the morning, restless sleep and morning headaches. Your GP has evaluation tools to assess whether or not you may be suffering from sleep apnoea.

> I recently discovered that I have severe sleep apnoea and I've been using a CPAP machine for the last month. The result is amazing so far. My energy levels improved so much. Brain fog, headaches, dry mouth no longer. So happy with my life again. I hardly recognise this new improved Catherine – she is back!
>
> – Catherine

Restless legs syndrome

A common sleep disorder in midlife is restless legs syndrome (RLS). Many women experience this – a painful feeling in the legs, or sometimes arms, that can feel like tingling or a deep itch. It's generally worse when lying down or sitting for an extended period of time, hence why it's so common at night-time. As the name suggests, your legs are restless and you have to keep moving them to feel relief. RLS can often happen in pregnancy too, but generally disappears after the baby is born. Low iron levels, diabetes or rheumatoid arthritis can also trigger RLS, so have these checked with your GP.

Reducing caffeine will help sleep in general and will also help RLS. Try having a warm bath with Epsom salts before bed, or a leg massage – you could add a magnesium body-oil spray to this, which may provide relief. Look to incorporate exercise into your daily routine, and if you are a smoker, try to stop the habit, as it's known to make this symptom and many others worse.

> Why does nobody talk about restless legs? This was hell for me. I dreaded going to bed, I knew I would wake in a few hours with my legs driving me nuts. And I just couldn't stop them moving, and I would lie there exhausted, close to tears and willing my legs to be calm. I am so grateful for the day I discovered magnesium – within one week they stopped and I got my sleep back.
>
> – Martina

Periodic limb movement disorder

Formerly called sleep myoclonus or nocturnal myoclonus, this disorder involves repetitive limb movements that happen during sleep and impact sleep quality.

SUPPLEMENTS

Some supplements that may help with sleep issues are:

- Magnesium powder, which is also excellent for the nervous system
- Valerian, lemon balm, chamomile, cherry powder (Morello cherry) and passionflower – helpful when you experience disturbed sleep
- 5-HTP, L-tryptophan and L-theanine may also improve sleep quality

MELATONIN

Your twenty-four-hour body clock uses melatonin to send messages to the brain indicating daytime and night-time. When it comes into operation, it's like a factory bell alerting everyone that the day is over – night is coming. Its job is to trigger the start of sleep – once you sleep, it starts to fall and dawn brings a stop to the production. Melatonin-containing foods include pistachios (unsalted), almonds, milk, tart cherries, oats, goji berries, eggs and salmon. Eating these during the day can help with melatonin production.

WHAT ELSE CAN HELP

- Relaxation techniques – practise the breathing exercise on page 262.
- Writing out your worries – if you are feeling anxious before bed, writing your worries down can help you get them out of your head. This is a great time to practise using a gratitude journal.
- HRT – many women experience an improvement in sleep when taking progesterone. (See Chapter 14 for more.)
- Sex – the bedroom is for two things: sleep and sex! Sex releases the hormone prolactin, which makes you calm, relaxed and primed for sleep.
- Over-the-counter sleep aids – these can be helpful in the short term but are not recommended for long-term use. If you are on medication there can be an interaction, so it is extremely important to seek medical advice before taking them.
- An evening cup of herbal tea like tulsi.

WHEN YOU CAN'T SLEEP

It's important not to let sleep, or the lack of it, become a stressor in your life. If you are someone who has been used to fewer hours of sleep over your life, then that may just be your own physical make-up. Remember, rest also brings benefits, so don't lie in bed worrying about not sleeping – a great step can be to read a book or just lie somewhere with dim lighting and listen to a meditation, and return to your bed when you feel sleepy. It's all about calmness and restfulness.

*   *   *

There is nothing better than waking up feeling rejuvenated and ready to go in the morning after a good night's sleep. I'm well aware of how difficult this may be during menopause, but it is deserving of our time, effort and attention so we can enjoy the finest night's sleep possible. Remember, this isn't simply to protect you through menopause: it's also to safeguard your brain and future health.

5

Genitourinary symptoms

Many of the symptoms of menopause ebb and flow over time, and we can often get a break from the intensity of symptoms by making tweaks to our lifestyle and/or medication. One symptom, though, does not get better with time unless we proactively take steps to address it. And one of the worst things about it is that we really don't talk about it *at all*. In my experience, women don't discuss this with their closest friends, and very often not even with their GP.

Pelvic-floor health and vaginal atrophy is a subject I have been very vocal about in my work, and it needs to be talked about more. It is a taboo within a taboo, if that is possible.

A few years back, I was chatting with a group of women about all aspects of menopause, and when I came to this topic, the room went quiet, heads went down and faces turned red. I know it's not comfortable. I wasn't rocking out to vagina tunes a few years ago myself, but now I will sing them from the hilltops to anyone who will listen! And that's because I have spoken to so many women who have been devastated by this aspect of menopause.

The good news is there are ample choices when it comes to treatment. And if you go to your GP and are told that sex is no longer part of your life or you should grin and bear it, then please change your GP.

I visited doctors, nurses, urologists, gynaecologists and clinics, including the sexual health clinic, in sheer desperation for someone to listen to me. I ended up for two years being treated for thrush, BV [bacterial vaginosis], herpes – in fact, anything but what had developed. I was not listened to. I was treated as if it was in my head and sent from pillar to post. At one point I told a doctor I did not want to go on any more and he ignored me. I left his surgery in tears and had a complete meltdown. I had reached a point in my life when I genuinely did not want to be in this world any more.

– Anonymous

THE GSM SYMPTOMS

The genitourinary syndrome of menopause (GSM), previously known as vaginal atrophy, encompasses many aspects of menopause that affect the vulva, vagina and urinary tract (including your bladder and urethra) due to the loss of oestrogen. The majority of menopausal symptoms will improve and lessen over time but the GSM symptoms will only worsen if left untreated.

WHAT IS VAGINAL DRYNESS?

Vaginal atrophy (atrophic vaginitis) is the thinning, drying and inflammation of the vaginal walls that can occur during perimenopause and menopause as oestrogen reserves decline. Vaginal atrophy is also referred to as vaginal dryness. With perimenopause comes a gradual decline in oestrogen – this has a direct impact on the tissues that respond to oestrogen, such as the tissues of the vagina and the vulva. The supply of oestrogen before perimenopause ensures the vaginal tissues are thick, moist and elastic. When the levels of oestrogen start to decline, these tissues become thinner, less elastic and more susceptible to friction and, in essence, are more easily injured. Think of oestrogen as your internal lubrication for all areas of your body. The drop in oestrogen reduces this much-needed lubrication and these changes can cause vaginal dryness, itchiness, UTIs (urinary tract infections), more frequent toilet breaks, painful smears, painful sex and many more symptoms. Fifty per cent of women will experience vaginal dryness in menopause. Unfortunately, treatment is often inadequate, despite how widespread the issue is.

What to look out for

- Bladder symptoms – urinating more often, stress incontinence (leakage), recurrent infections (UTIs), uncomfortable compared to before
- Discomfort during sex
- Smear tests more uncomfortable than before
- Bleeding outside your period with or without sex
- Itching – please do not self-diagnose as thrush unless you have checked and see visible signs of thrush
- Vulval burning/inflammation
- Watery vaginal discharge
- Bladder, bowel or uterine prolapse – this can be felt by a bulging sensation in the vaginal walls
- Vaginal infections – as the acid balance changes you can be more susceptible to these

TREATMENT OPTIONS

See your doctor

First of all, open up about your symptoms – many women feel shy discussing this condition. Talk to your GP – don't self-diagnose. Your GP should then perform a pelvic exam, during which they examine your pelvic organs, external genitalia, vagina and cervix. They may also check for signs of pelvic organ prolapse – this is manifested by bulges in the walls of your vagina from your bladder or bowel or through loss of the support tissues of the uterus. A urine test may also be taken if you have urinary symptoms. Some doctors may also do an acid balance test, which involves taking a sample of vaginal fluids or placing a paper indicator strip into your vagina to test its acid balance.

The doctor performs this to rule out the following:

- Local vaginal infection – for example, bacterial vaginosis, trichomonas (a common sexually transmitted disease), candidiasis and endometritis (inflammation of the uterine lining). Infections like these can occur at the same time as vaginal atrophy, as it predisposes the vagina to bacterial infection.

- Other causes of vaginal bleeding or post-menopausal bleeding.
- Unchecked diabetes, which can cause vaginal or urinary symptoms.
- Vaginal irritation caused by certain soaps, toilet wipes, panty liners, spermicides, condoms, poorly formulated lubricants, biological washing powder or tight-fitting clothes.

It's a good idea to familiarise yourself with your vulva (the vulva is external; your vagina is internal and cannot be seen). We have become very good at checking our breasts on a regular basis, but this self-check needs to extend to the vulva so you know how it looks and can see if changes occur. I would encourage you to take a mirror, look and become familiar with your vulva.

Moisturisers

A vaginal moisturiser will hydrate the tissues and is an essential step. It can provide immediate relief for dryness and also help with cell repair. Ideally, it should be part of your regular routine, just like you moisturise your face. And more importantly, it is a key ingredient in future-proofing your long-term health. It doesn't just protect your vaginal health but also your bladder and urinary health.

When buying a moisturiser, please take the time to look at the ingredients, as you are putting this into your body – select a moisturiser with good-quality ingredients and ensure it is unperfumed. The best time to use it is at bedtime. The effects of moisturisers are longer lasting than lubricants, generally two to three days. Apply them regularly for optimum benefit.

Hyaluronic acid is already present naturally in the vagina and helps with hydration and elasticity. Using moisturisers containing hyaluronic acid may provide instant relief from feelings of dryness, itching and inflammation.

If you have no symptoms of vaginal atrophy but are concerned about an upcoming smear test, a good tip is to start moisturising daily seven days prior to the test, then stop for the two days just before it (to ensure it doesn't impact the results). If you have ongoing symptoms, you should work out a treatment plan with your GP or gynaecologist and, ideally, aim to have your smear after about four to six weeks of local oestrogen.

Lubricants

Lubricants are designed specifically for intercourse, to reduce any friction and ensure comfort. They are similar to vaginal moisturisers but have shorter action. They will be absorbed more quickly if you are very dry, so this is where the moisturiser adds more value. With lubricants and moisturisers, I always advise to do a patch test on your body externally before applying internally – we can all react differently to ingredients.

Lubricants come in several forms: water-, oil-, silicone- and natural-oil-based. Any water-based product has to contain preservatives for stability – some women can be sensitive to certain ingredients so it is important to find what works best for you and suits your body. Oil-based lubricants cannot be used with condoms; only water-based lubricants can. Please also note the difference between mineral oils and natural plant-based or vegetable oils. Baby oil and Vaseline are by-products of refined petroleum oil and are not recommended here. Silicone does not occur naturally in the body and does not let the skin do what it should do naturally – in my view, it's not ideal to put into your vagina, but some people prefer it. Lubricants that contain glycerine and glycols have been linked to outbreaks of thrush so always check the ingredients. Look out, too, for the pH of the lubricant – ideally you are looking for a range of 3.5 to 5, which is similar to the pH of the vaginal tissues.

If you're having local oestrogen treatment (see below), it's a personal choice whether to use a moisturiser and/or lubricant. It is fine to use a lubricant when you are using local oestrogen but it's best to use a moisturiser on a different day to the local oestrogen.

When having sex, remember, the more slippery the better: this will prevent friction for you. I would suggest applying an oil-based lubricant on yourself first – this will protect the tissues. Then apply a water-based lubricant on your partner or any toys you are using. These are just suggestions, of course – you will need to find what works best for you and your partner. And remember, orgasms with or without your partner are very helpful. They provide essential blood flow to the area.

Lubricants are for the short term, to avoid any friction from sexual activity. Moisturisers provide much-needed moisture to the vaginal walls. Think lubricant short-term, moisturiser long-term health.

Hormone replacement therapy (HRT)

Discuss with your GP about using local or systemic oestrogen therapy – both are highly effective and will improve the symptoms of GSM. (See Chapter 14 for more on systemic HRT). If you have only GSM symptoms, then local therapy to the affected area will be the first-line treatment. This is helpful in restoring vaginal elasticity, promoting the bacteria of the vagina, increasing genital blood flow and reducing dryness and dyspareunia (painful sex). If you are concerned about using HRT, please know a year's supply of local oestrogen is equal to one tablet of the lowest HRT dose. To date, no research has shown any risks associated with local oestrogen.

Local oestrogen comes in two types, oestradiol and oestriol, and in the following forms:

- Vaginal ring – for example, Estring. This is a soft, flexible ring you can insert yourself into the upper part of the vagina. It needs to be replaced every three months, as it releases a daily dose of oestradiol over ninety days.
- Vaginal cream – for example, Estrace (oral form also available) or Ovestin. These are inserted via applicator at night-time (or as prescribed by your

GP). Standard dose is one applicator up to the marker (0.5mg oestriol in 0.5g of cream) a day for the first two to three weeks (at most four weeks). Then the dose is one applicator up to the marker twice a week.

• Vaginal pessary – Vagifem is an oestrogen tablet inserted via an applicator; Vagirux is a more environmentally friendly option, with a non-plastic applicator; Imvaggis, a lower-dose alternative, is a pessary inserted without an applicator so may suit those who find using applicators uncomfortable. Dosage is similar to the vaginal cream.

Local oestrogen essentially provides a signal to the body to hydrate the area. Generally, women find improvements within a few weeks of starting treatment.

If you have ongoing uterine bleeding or active breast cancer, you will not be able to use local oestrogen. If you are using tamoxifen, you will need to consult with your oncologist before starting local treatment.

If you have undergone cancer treatment and your form of cancer indicates that you cannot use local oestrogen like Vagifem, then the first-line treatment is a non-hormonal vaginal moisturiser. It is important this product does not contain parabens (see Resources for recommendations). I would also recommend using omega-7. If you find using a vaginal moisturiser does not bring relief, talk to your GP about alternative supports.

Vaginal DHEA

The adrenal glands produce DHEA, an androgen. DHEA is a large source of sex steroid hormones after menopause. A recent addition to the medical support for GSM is a pessary known as Intrarosa – the DHEA it contains converts into oestrogen and progesterone in the vagina.

Ospemifene

This medication is used for treating dyspareunia (painful sex) due to GSM. It is used when local oestrogen is contraindicated. It helps the vaginal lining with a minimal impact on the endometrial tissue. However, it can cause an increase in hot flushes.

Laser therapy

This can help to improve blood flow and encourage the production of collagen, all of which will help the support, elasticity and lubrication of the vaginal area. Be warned: there are several different forms of laser therapy, and some ablative laser treatments can be harmful. Non-ablative erbium laser therapy has proven safety and efficacy when provided by an expert practitioner. It is very important to see a specialist physiotherapist or doctor to confirm a diagnosis before you consider what treatment is likely to help your problem. Do your research and ensure you are attending a professional who is well versed in this area.

Natural oils and vitamins

Sea buckthorn oil: Omega-7 comes from sea buckthorn, a berry bush naturally found in Asia and Europe. Ongoing studies show that sea buckthorn can help maintain the health and integrity of the mucous membranes in the vagina and can be very helpful for women who may not be able to use local HRT. It has been used in Asian traditional medicine for over a thousand years and is good for the immune system in general because of its antioxidant content. It also contains vitamin A, which is good for the health of your mucous membranes. This will help with dry eyes and dry mouth symptoms too. If you are experiencing vaginal dryness, it may help, and it can be taken in addition to HRT.

Natural oils: Many women find extra virgin coconut oil, vitamin E oil and almond oil to be beneficial as moisturisers and lubricants, though they are not regulated for this use and can vary in quality. (Note that they cannot be used with latex condoms.) Coconut oil comes with the added benefit of having antibacterial qualities; however, this can have a flip side, as it can affect your vaginal microbiome.

Vitamin D: This is crucial in menopause, and many people have to take it as a supplement, as we do not get enough sunshine in Ireland! Current research indicates it can be effective in helping vaginal dryness – this is based on using a vaginal suppository and, unfortunately, I have not found such a product available in Europe. But I would highly recommend taking an oral vitamin D spray, as this is essential for overall immune health.

Omega-3 and zinc are also beneficial in alleviating dryness.

Dilators

Vaginal dilators can be a good addition to your treatment plan for vaginal atrophy. They are graded very small to large and can benefit you in several ways. If you are undergoing cancer treatment or pelvic radiotherapy where potentially there can be damage to local tissues, using a dilator will help prevent scarring and contraction of these tissues (discuss with your oncologist). If you are experiencing painful sex, your body may begin to anticipate the pain and the muscles of the vagina contract – this becomes a cycle of fear, contraction and pain. A graded dilator will help retrain the body to understand that this isn't painful and it puts you in control. Dilators can also be useful before a smear test if you are anxious about it or not sexually active. Silicone dilators are best and it is important to cover them with lubricant. Where possible, it is beneficial to use these under the guidance of a physiotherapist specialising in women's health.

I had breast cancer, and my vaginal dryness is off the scale – what can I do?

If you have undergone cancer treatment and your form of cancer indicates that you cannot use local oestrogen like Vagifem, the first-line treatment is a non-hormonal vaginal moisturiser. It is important that this product does not contain parabens. Omega-7 may also be beneficial. If you find using a non-hormonal vaginal moisturiser does not bring relief, talk to your GP about alternative supports.

Personal choices

Your vagina may need extra moisturiser and/or lubricant, but remember that what you use is a matter of personal choice. Many women report different success with a wide variety of products so it can be a case of trial and error until you find what works for you. Some other choices you can make:

- Smoking reduces blood circulation and your vaginal area needs a good blood flow, so if you smoke, do try to stop.
- Avoid perfumed toilet paper and sanitary pads.
- Avoid internal douches/washes – water alone is perfect!
- Tight clothing may be uncomfortable – try switching to looser clothing until you have got a handle on the issue.

Conditions to be aware of

Lichen sclerosus: a skin condition that creates patchy white regions, most often seen in the genital or anal areas. Mild cases may show no symptoms; moderate to severe cases may involve redness, itching, tearing, bleeding and pain during sex. Post-menopausal women are most likely to be affected by this condition, as hormone imbalances are a suspected cause. If there is any doubt about the diagnosis, ask to be referred to a vulval dermatologist. In rare cases, this condition can lead to vulval cancer, so it is important to get a correct diagnosis and treatment with local steroids.

Lichen planus: an autoimmune condition that attacks the skin, hair, nails and mucous membranes. It can look different depending on where it appears. In the mouth and vaginal area, lichen planus can look like white lacy patches and is sometimes accompanied by painful sores. On the skin, lichen planus presents as itchy purplish bumps, most commonly on the wrist and forearm. Ask your GP to refer you to a dermatologist specialising in this area.

Dyspareunia: a clinical word for painful sex. This can be caused by physical factors, like lack of lubrication, or emotional factors, like depression or anxiety.

Frequently, negative tension in the pelvic floor muscles is a factor as well. Certain medical conditions like endometriosis and uterine fibroids can also cause pain during intercourse. The first step is ruling out vaginal atrophy with your GP, who can then point you in the right direction.

Vaginismus: involuntary spasms of the vaginal wall triggered by fear or anxiety that prevent anything being inserted into the vagina. Frequently, there is an underlying condition associated with this pain reaction. It is important to know that this is not just you reacting without a reason. Treatments include psychosexual therapy, relaxation techniques and pelvic floor exercises.

Vulvodynia: pain around the vulva that can cause discomfort during sex or while sitting for long periods. The cause is unknown, but there is always a sensitivity of the nerves at the entrance to the vagina. Associated factors include increased muscle tone in the pelvic floor, hormonal changes, endometriosis, inflammatory bowel disorders and there is a hereditary link too. You should talk to your GP if this is something you're worried about.

THE URINARY SIDE OF THINGS

I have spoken with hundreds of women who were told that experiencing urinary issues of all kinds is a normal part of getting older and they should just accept it and 'move on'. This should never be the case. Common issues in this area are:

- Recurring UTIs
- Various forms of incontinence
- Passing urine more often during the day and at night
- Pelvic organ prolapse

Bladder health

Earlier I mentioned the opportunities menopause brings to prepare ourselves for optimum health in our later years. Bladder health is a non-negotiable part of that. There is a well-choreographed, synchronised arrangement between the nervous system, your brain, bladder, urethra and pelvic floor muscles. And this is a dance where things can go wrong as we go through menopause. The key is frequently, but not always, the pelvic floor and I would urge you, when you think of exercise, to include this in your daily routine. Exercising it will help maintain good bladder function and also a healthy sex life. Let's be honest, as you're reading this you're probably thinking, 'Oh god, I should be doing those exercises.' Chances are you're not doing them regularly – and doing them right is just as important. One in three women experience pelvic floor dysfunction.

The pelvic floor muscle is like a sling that attaches to the pelvic bones. Its role is to control bladder and bowel function. It also plays a supportive role by holding your bladder, bowel and uterus in place. The pelvic floor can come under pressure due to pregnancy, childbirth, excess weight, chronic coughing, ongoing constipation, vigorous activity and menopause. In menopause, as oestrogen levels change, the pelvic floor weakens and it is less elastic. This can result in various forms of incontinence:

- Stress incontinence – when your bladder is under pressure from an activity you are doing, for example, a cough, a sneeze or lifting something
- Urinary incontinence – an uncontrollable loss of urine
- Urinary urgency/overactive bladder – a sudden urge to urinate even when the bladder is not full
- Urge incontinence – a sudden urge to urinate that cannot wait
- Overflow incontinence – urinary leakage that occurs when the bladder is too full
- Mixed incontinence – a combination of urge and stress incontinence
- Nocturia – frequent waking in the night because of the need to urinate
- Anal incontinence – lack of control over bowel movements or flatulence

The time to work on your pelvic floor is right now: there is no reason to wait.

Chronic bladder issues will impact all parts of your life and your work if you start to experience them.

> I never knew there was such a thing as a specialist physio who looked after the more intimate part of my health. It has been an eye-opener for me and has made my pelvic floor exercises a priority now in my day. I was going every few months as I was leaking, and now things are so much better, I am not wearing a pad any more which I am so happy about. I think so many women think it's normal as we get older to leak. It's not.
>
> – Carol

Key steps to take for bladder health:

- Engage with a women's health physiotherapist. This is the very first place to start. A physical examination is usually part of the process and will give you a great understanding of how your body is adjusting physically to the changes in this area. They will also ensure you understand how to perform your pelvic floor exercises properly.
- Access online guides and tutorials that will talk you through pelvic floor exercises (see Resources).
- Train your bladder – only go to the toilet when you need to. The bladder can get used to bad habits and it is important to train it to behave when you step out of the house. But do go regularly – don't hold on until you really need to go, and when you do go, take your time and don't rush it.
- If you play sports, I would highly recommend wearing pelvic support shorts (see Resources).
- Drink plenty of water to ensure you keep hydrated – even if you have symptoms in this area, this is not the time to stop drinking water. It is important to ensure regular urination to avoid any infections.
- Weight management – we want to put less pressure on the bladder, so this is a good reason to work on daily eating habits and manage your weight.

- Avoid constipation (see Chapter 19) – this will put further pressure on your bladder.
- Be mindful of your caffeine and alcohol intake – these can irritate your bladder. Both are diuretics that will make you urinate more.

Urinary tract infections (UTIs)

UTIs are very common in menopause and can become a vicious cycle, as they're treated with antibiotics, which can sometimes result in thrush and impact vaginal dryness. Through menopause and ageing, the urethra (the tube that takes urine from your bladder to the toilet) can become thinner and weaken. The vaginal microbiome (bacteria) is also changing, which can compound this issue further.

Supports to investigate:

- Local oestrogen, as described earlier
- D-mannose supplements – these can help prevent UTIs
- Antibiotics
- Vitamin A, vitamin C, magnesium

Pelvic organ prolapse

This occurs when the pelvic organs drop and create a bulge in the vagina or anus. According to women's health physiotherapist Maeve Whelan, 11 per cent of women will undergo surgery due to prolapse. Similar to vaginal atrophy, this is rarely discussed, but it should be. Many symptoms women believe are due to digestives issues (especially flatulence and constipation) may well be related to prolapse. There are various forms of prolapse and a physical examination is the first step to take. Symptoms of a prolapse are as follows:

- Feeling or seeing a bulge in your vaginal or anal area. It may feel worse after standing for long periods or when you go to sit down.

- A feeling that your bladder doesn't empty fully when you go to the toilet.
- More frequent toilet visits.
- Flatulence – 10 per cent of women have issues controlling stool or wind.
- Recurring UTIs.
- Constipation.
- Lower back pain.

The treatment is generally the use of a vaginal ring pessary that helps support the vaginal organs. It is key here to work with a women's health physiotherapist to investigate other treatment options. Surgery may also be considered.

Can I take any medications to help with my bladder symptoms?

Anticholinergic medications may be prescribed for an overactive bladder; when these cannot be tolerated there is another drug called Mirabegron. See also the non-hormonal options in Chapter 14. (For more information on bladder health, see Resources.)

* * *

At a recent Menopause Success Summit I held, we had a lively discussion about vaginal dryness. As a taboo within a taboo that we are working to shatter, we really need to open this discussion. Just as we moisturise our hands and face, it is a good habit to moisturise your vulva and your vagina on a regular basis. Being proactive is the way forward – 'prevention is better than cure'. Your long-term sexual and bladder health will thank you.

6

Let's talk about sex

There is no more complex and controversial subject, I believe, than sexual health – from roundabout talks about the birds and the bees and the whispered conversations of childhood about how babies are made, to the guilt you can feel if you have been raised with the view of sex as a bad thing or the trauma of abuse that you may, unfortunately, have experienced.

According to the World Health Organisation (WHO), sexual health is 'a state of physical, emotional, mental and social well-being related to sexuality; not merely the absence of dysfunction or infirmity', and they describe female sexuality as a basic human right, as well as an important part of women's physical health.

Do you remember the swirls in your tum when you first kissed someone – maybe it was during the slow set at the local disco or in your local park? Then the mounting desire that came as you progressed through puberty – the desire that maybe took just seconds to build – the intensity of passion. And then as the years progressed came more fuel to the flame.

Menopause: the ice bucket thrown on any vestige of passion!

The good news is you can rekindle it – it just takes more time, thought and consideration. It is crucial we become more comfortable talking about this aspect of menopause and its closely aligned sister – vaginal symptoms.

Loss of libido affects 69 per cent of women – and this may impact your partner and relationships too. And relationships and support are vital as you navigate the choppy waters of menopause. Of course, not everyone will experience this loss of libido, and, in fact, some can even return to those early sun-kissed days of adolescence.

> For my forties, I endured severe vaginal dryness, making intercourse almost unbearable. I had bleeding after sex, and the pain and discomfort meant I didn't enjoy our sexual connection and grew to dread it.
>
> – Anonymous

SEX DOESN'T STOP WHEN YOU HIT FIFTY

Several years ago I met a woman who had been advised by her doctor to just accept that the chapter of her life that involved sex was closed. At the time, she was experiencing vaginal dryness and sex was very painful for her. She was fifty-three and devastated. Sex does not stop when you hit fifty! Please do not accept this ageist view of sexual health, and ensure you get the treatment you need if you are experiencing painful sex (see Chapter 5).

Yes, if you are suffering sleep issues, exhaustion and drenching night sweats you may not feel in the mood for sex, but that will pass. Alternatively, you might be quite glad that this chapter is closed for you. An early night in bed with a good book can often be more tempting than intimacy. It is individual and unique to you.

In chatting with a doctor recently, I asked when she thought the foreplay/build-up to sex starts in these years. She reckoned a week prior – I reckon it's two! As we get older it can be more difficult to just switch from the daily routines of work, parenthood and chores to thinking about your sex life. It requires planning, thought and making it a priority in your life.

It's also important to remember that even in menopause you can be prone to sexually transmitted diseases; you can, of course, still have casual sex, and if so, you need to protect yourself against STIs.

HOW YOUR SEXUAL HEALTH CAN IMPACT YOUR LIFE

It's not just about the bedroom: sexual health affects you emotionally and psychologically; it affects your mental and physical health and, importantly, your self-esteem. The most common symptoms impacting sexual health are low desire, poor lubrication, vaginal dryness, dyspareunia (pain during sex), stress, anxiety and depression.

It's imperative to pay attention to what your body is feeling – don't hide away from physical discomfort if it exists. There are many treatment options that can be investigated.

Some medications can also affect your libido, so it is important to understand any possible side effects of the medications you are taking. Antidepressants, beta-blockers, sleep medications and others can have an impact. Underlying medical conditions can also be a cause – for example, a thyroid imbalance that is not treated successfully.

LIBIDO AND MENOPAUSE

Not every woman will experience changes in her sex life in menopause, but the majority will at some stage. The psychological aspects of menopause may make you feel irritable and simply 'not in the mood'. And sleep issues due to night sweats won't make you feel like a goddess in the bedroom. Changing hormone levels can result in vaginal atrophy, making sex painful and uncomfortable, and this may also lower your sex drive, which results in taking you longer to get aroused.

Of course, being less interested in sex as you get older is not necessarily a medical condition – it can simply be life and age and your individual attitude to sex. Please don't feel you have to engage in sex to satisfy your partner – this should never be the case. I have met women with severe vaginal dryness who went through very painful intercourse to 'keep their partners happy'. This is *not* OK.

If you are unhappy with your sexual health, please talk to a trusted source like your GP, a women's health physiotherapist or a sex therapist for support (see Resources).

When you feel like your libido is not as you would like it to be, the first things to consider are:

- Current medications
- Underlying medical conditions
- Stress in your life, your emotional health at any specific time
- The health of your relationship with your partner or with yourself (how comfortable you are with self-pleasure)

GOOD REASONS TO HAVE SEX

If you are comfortable with it, it really can be worth creating time and space for sex in your life – the benefits are far-reaching.

Better vaginal health

Sex improves vaginal lubrication, genital blood flow and even vaginal suppleness. It can increase your libido, causing you to crave sex more frequently, ensuring that your vaginal health is optimised. Regular enjoyable sex and orgasms can also aid sleep, particularly when getting a decent night's sleep might be difficult. And frequent orgasms and the use of a sex toy can help you maintain your sexual health, irrespective of age or gender or whether you have a partner.

Release of the feel-good hormone

Oxytocin is a brain-produced hormone that promotes an overall sensation of well-being and happiness. While sex and orgasms can boost oxytocin levels, a plain old hug with your partner can do the trick as well. Oxytocin is known as the love hormone, as it aids in the formation of bonds, the development of trust and the deepening of intimacy between people. High oxytocin levels can result in a more positive attitude to life, which leads to increased self-esteem.

Mood boost

It's all too easy to bury our head in the pillow and attempt to ignore the world when we're tired, but consciously waking up early for a morning interlude can put you in a good mood for the rest of the day. This is because sex can boost the creation of serotonin, the natural mood stabiliser connected to happiness.

Lower blood pressure

Enjoyable sex improves our mood by lowering stress levels, which has a positive effect on our blood pressure.

An immune shot

Regular intercourse has been related to higher levels of immunoglobulin A (IgA), an antibody that can protect you against colds and other diseases.

A skip in your step

Sex releases endorphins, which are natural painkillers that can also boost our motivation levels. When we're feeling lethargic, it's easy to make excuses not to exercise; however, if our bodies are naturally motivated by endorphins, we're more likely to make the time to exercise and be more productive.

That afterglow

Oxytocin also has anti-inflammatory properties that aid in skin-cell healing. Sex increases oestrogen levels, which improves skin elasticity and hydration. Our circulation is increased, which gives you that afterglow.

SEXUAL WELL-BEING IN MENOPAUSE

Do we take much time to think of our sexual health? Life is busy and complicated enough as it is. It is also very personal, and we all have different views and attitudes toward sex. I have chatted with women who have abstained from sex for years, others for months and others who have a regular habit in place with their partner or with themselves. There is no right answer here. But as with many things in life, if you can put more effort and time into it, you will reap the rewards.

Self-pleasure

For many of us, masturbation was never discussed growing up and was considered a bad thing. But try thinking of sex as a basic human right, once it's consensual and pain free, and this is a step toward understanding that you can and should masturbate. You should feel totally guilt free and comfortable doing this. It is healthy and normal: fact.

And apart from the pleasurable aspect, there are health benefits, too, of masturbation – chiefly, blood flow to the vulva and vagina, keeping it toned, and a swift release of feel-good endorphins, which help reduce stress and encourage sleep.

Talk to your partner

Let's be honest: it's not easy to open a conversation about sex with your partner, but it is essential. Communication is key here. Getting older and experiencing chronic health problems like heart disease or diabetes can affect your sexual health and how you feel about sex. This impacts not only you but also your partner on a physical and emotional level. If you are finding sex painful, you must tell your partner – if they are unaware, they cannot help. An understanding partner will want to support you to resolve how you are feeling.

A good tip is to *not* have a conversation about sex in the bedroom: find a neutral spot that isn't associated with it – go for a walk, sit in the garden and so on. Some possible topics to discuss include:

- What feels good and what doesn't
- Times that you may feel more relaxed
- Which positions are more comfortable

- Whether you need more time to get aroused than before
- Concerns you have about the way your appearance may be changing
- Ways to enjoy physical connection other than vaginal intercourse, such as oral sex or massage

Building up to sexual intimacy can happen in the small details of everyday life – the nice things, the small gestures your partner does for you. And having time to reconnect with each other is all part of building desire and communication. So book that nice restaurant, go for a long hike – whatever it is you enjoy doing together. 'Couplepause' is a phrase used to emphasise the importance of working *together* as sexual health changes with age – not separately.

Counselling

Sexual counselling, CBT and couples counselling can be of great benefit. Past trauma therapy can be life transforming at this stage if this has not already happened and issues are still being felt from the past (see Chapter 12 for more).

Sex toys

These can be a great addition to your sex life, and there is a vast array to choose from – chatting to a knowledgeable resource in this area can be helpful to decide which might work for you (see Resources). Some key types include:

- Simple bullet vibrators – these are a great starting point.
- Clitoral stimulators – 70 per cent of women need clitoral stimulation to achieve an orgasm and cannot orgasm through penetration alone.
- Air pulse/sonic wave toys – these have transformed orgasm for countless people.
- Toys for your partner.
- Specific toys for partners with erectile issues who may be avoiding sex as a result.

As we get older, sex changes for us and 'sexploration' is important – what satisfied you in the past may not today. Many women feel freer now to discover what works best for them. It may be a combination of more body confidence, more time or children leaving home that opens a new chapter in your sex life.

PRACTICAL STEPS

Your sexual health is inextricably linked to the health and vibrancy of your life. Here are some practical steps you can take to ensure this remains a pleasurable and fulfilling part of your life during and after menopause.

- Address any pain during or related to sex, like vaginal atrophy.
- Introduce moisturisers and lubricants – this is essential.
- Make annual appointments with your women's health physiotherapist and practise your exercises! These will strengthen your pelvic muscles, which are part of reaching an orgasm, and help blood flow to the area (see Chapter 5).
- Get regular exercise – physical activity will help your mood and energy levels and keep you healthy and fit. These will all help your sexual desire.
- The 6 Ms of menopause (see Chapters 17 to 22) are all important here too, as more energy and good mental health are key components of good sexual health.
- Make sex and/or self-pleasure a regular in your life – this will increase blood flow to the vaginal area and help keep tissues healthy.
- Eliminate smoking – it can reduce blood flow to the vaginal area and lower the effects of oestrogen, making arousal more difficult.
- Talk to your doctor if you are concerned about your sexual health.

THE ROLE OF TESTOSTERONE

As we saw in Chapter 1, this hormone is just as important to women as it is to men. It contributes to libido, arousal and the ability to reach orgasm by its impact on dopamine levels. Adding testosterone to your HRT regime may be considered where there are ongoing libido, energy, brain fog and low-mood symptoms. However, at the time of writing, the only clinical indication for prescribing testosterone is for low sexual desire, based on current guidance from NICE (National Institute for Health and Care Excellence) and the British Menopause Society.

If you are starting testosterone, it is not required that your doctor measure your current levels, but this is definitely good information to have. That way, after a few months, you will be able to see what impact it is having, not just by looking at symptoms but also by understanding what is being absorbed and used in your body. If your levels are already high, you may not want to add more into your body. It is good practice to check your blood pressure and know your cholesterol levels prior to treatment.

Currently, there are no licensed female testosterone products – the product you will receive is a male version that can be used for women. The most common forms are Androfeme, a testosterone cream, and Testogel. The gel or cream should be applied to clean, dry skin, ideally on the stomach area or upper thigh. I would recommend the upper inner thigh, as you may experience hair growth in the area of application. Ensure it dries before dressing, and wash your hands thoroughly. Do not wash the application area for two to three hours after applying.

Clinical trials showed that two-thirds of women responded well to testosterone, but the response is not always immediate: it can take eight to twelve weeks to take effect. If you are taking it, be prepared to commit to three to six months before seeing a change. If there is no change after this time, discuss the next steps with your doctor. An annual review with your doctor is also recommended to look at symptom management and the latest research on testosterone so that you are informed about the risks and benefits at any given time.

The trick with testosterone is getting the dosage right, as different women will report different experiences. Watch out for the following and discuss with your doctor if they occur:

- Prominent increased body hair at site of application – this is common, so look at spreading it more thinly, changing where you apply it and discuss reducing dosage.
- Hair loss, acne and hirsutism throughout the body – these are uncommon effects.
- Deepening of the voice and enlarged clitoris – these are rare effects.
- The standard rules of HRT administration apply in relation to when it should be avoided (see Chapter 14), with the addition of, if you are an elite athlete, ensuring the testosterone levels are maintained within the standard female range.

CONTRACEPTION – WHY YOU STILL NEED IT

Yes, the likelihood of conceiving drops when you are aged forty-five to fifty, but there is still a 10 per cent chance. And while you might be having longer cycles, you can still ovulate and still get pregnant. The general medical advice is that contraception can be stopped one year after your periods stop if this occurs over the age of fifty. If you reach menopause before the age of fifty, it should be continued for two years after your last period. At the age of fifty-five you can stop contraception if you are still having the odd period, as the risk of pregnancy is very low. Your doctor can advise based on your personal situation and medical history. And don't forget, HRT is not a form of contraception!

* * *

Feeling exhausted, stressed and hot will not help your appetite for sex. But if you look at your sexual health as another aspect of your menopause that needs attention, now and for the future, then you may start to prioritise it more and realise that, if you wish, it can be another invigorating aspect of your life now, where you know what you like and have the confidence to communicate it.

7

Bone health

We need to look after and strengthen our bones in the menopause years. This is an essential step in protecting our long-term health – being active and fit in your later years is all about what you do now.

In 2019, statistics showed that 32 million Europeans were diagnosed with osteoporosis, 25.5 million of whom were women. According to the Irish Osteoporosis Society (IOS), it's estimated that 50 per cent of women in Ireland over fifty have osteoporosis, but only 19 per cent are diagnosed. Globally, osteoporosis causes more than 8.9 million fractures annually, resulting in an osteoporosis fracture every three seconds, and one in three women over the age of fifty will experience osteoporosis fractures. Hip (70 per cent) and forearm (80 per cent) fractures are the most common. If you have had one vertebral fracture (broken bone in your back), this increases your risk of a new vertebral fracture in the following year.

Your bones are not just 'calcified tubes'. They continue to change and adapt as we go through life. Women are at peak bone health at about thirty years of age and then decline starts. The chief bone-forming years are in adolescence, and not many of us think about bone health in those years. But all is not lost: there is much we can do to protect our bones and prevent further deterioration as we age.

WHAT HAPPENS TO OUR BONES AS WE AGE?

Many of us don't realise how alive and constantly active our bones are – maybe we look at bone replicas or skeletons on TV and think that bones are fixed structures. The reality is very different. Bone is a living tissue that is constantly being removed and replaced throughout life. As we age, there is gradual increase in bone loss, but this increases significantly in women during menopause due to the loss of oestrogen – about half of a woman's lifetime bone loss occurs in the first ten years after menopause.

What are the signs or symptoms of declining bone health?

This is a silent disease. There are no early warning signs. A diagnosis is confirmed by having a DXA scan or an injury (which may trigger a DXA scan). The hip, spine and wrist bones are the most common areas of injury where fractures (broken bones) occur. Back pain, loss of height or change in body shape and unexplained broken bones are signs of osteoporosis.

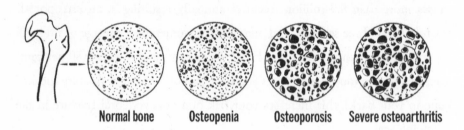

Normal bone   Osteopenia   Osteoporosis   Severe osteoarthritis

OSTEOPENIA

This is the precursor to osteoporosis and, as such, puts you at high risk of developing osteoporosis – it is the early stages of bone loss. However, research shows that the majority of fractures occur in the moderate to marked osteopenia range. This is a stark warning to up your game and take action about your bone health, by having the causes of your bone loss investigated and addressed, not assumed.

OSTEOPOROSIS

This occurs when your bones become weak and fragile, increasing your risk of breaking a bone, even with a minor fall. Many people assume that they will know if they are losing bone, but no one feels bone loss or bone strength improving. Fractures can have a detrimental impact, not just causing pain but often resulting in loss of independence and premature death. This is why it is vital to make your bone health a priority, as research shows most fractures are preventable. Some of the two hundred risk factors that place a person at risk of developing osteoporosis are:

- Early menopause – under the age of forty-five
- Family history of osteoporosis and/or osteopenia
- Late onset of periods – if your periods started after the age of fifteen you are at higher risk
- History of pre-menstrual tension (PMT)
- Endometriosis
- Hysterectomy
- Your ethnic background – Caucasians and Asians are highest risk
- Your body type – a thin frame if you are underweight for your height
- Rheumatoid arthritis
- Sedentary lifestyle
- Smoking
- High stress levels
- Frequent and high caffeine and/or alcohol use
- Overtraining
- Anorexia or bulimia, overtraining, or a combination of two or more
- Overactive thyroid or overactive parathyroid
- Low vitamin D, which is very common in Ireland due to the lack of sunshine and foods containing vitamin D
- Diabetes

- Certain medications – for example, the contraceptive Depo-Provera has been shown to cause bone loss
- Certain treatments such as chemotherapy, radiation and Arimidex
- Use of steroids/glucocorticoids – for example, prednisone or cortisone

How is it treated?

Treatment will be targeted at either helping to prevent bone loss or increasing bone formation, which reduces your risk of fractures. Your doctor or consultant will assess the best route, based on your DXA results, the cause(s) of your bone loss, your age and medical history. In order for you to improve your bone health, it is essential that your causes of bone loss are investigated and addressed. Treatments may include bisphosphonates, SERMs (selective oestrogen receptor modulators), injections that are six-monthly, or daily for severe bone loss, and once-yearly intravenous (IVs). The contraceptive pill or individualised HRT may also be considered especially, where an eating disorder co-exists in pre-menopause years. For those with early menopause, HRT is an important part of long-term treatment.

To date, no large-scale studies have been completed which compare HRT to other medical treatments for osteopososis. HRT can be an effective treatment where both osteoporosis and menopause symptoms exist.

THE DXA SCAN

A DXA scan (sometimes called DEXA) is a type of medical imaging test. It uses very low levels of radiation to measure how strong your bones are. DXA stands for 'dual-energy X-ray absorptiometry'. If you have heard that a DXA scan contains significant radiation, this is not accurate: it contains 10 per cent of the radiation of a regular chest X-ray. Flying from Dublin to New York may expose you to more radiation than a DXA scan. Measuring bone density tells you how much mineral is in your bone: this is your bone mass. You lie on your back for ten to fifteen minutes while a bar moves back and forth above you.

If you have early menopause, as soon as it is diagnosed, no matter what your age, a DXA scan is the first step you should take. Remember that osteoporosis is commonly thought of as an 'old woman's disease', therefore you will need to be proactive. It is much cheaper, less painful and certainly less stressful to prevent fractures than to treat them and live with the secondary consequences of them.

For natural menopause, it is a crucial step. You may have had risk factors for bone loss prior to your menopause, and already have lost bone. It is very important that, if your DXA scan shows bone loss, a plan to prevent further bone loss is put in place: it is very rare that a person cannot improve their bone health.

The results of your DXA scan will refer to T scores. These compare your results to an average thirty-year-old woman, as this is the average age of peak bone density.

You may hear about Z scores, especially if you have early menopause. This compares your reading to your own age group and is most commonly used for children and adolescents.

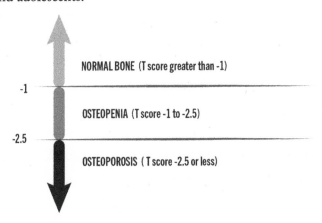

How often should you repeat a DXA scan?

If your initial DXA results are good, that is great news. However, it does not automatically mean you are in the clear. Any woman going through menopause will lose bone, some more than others.

The IOS recommend that women going through menopause have a DXA scan annually, even if the first one is negative for bone loss. Since no one knows which women will lose a significant amount of bone, it is cheaper to have a scan than pay for fractures that could have been prevented.

Many people are unaware that breaking bones can be life altering:

- 20 per cent of people aged sixty-plus who fracture their hip will pass away within six to twelve months.
- 50 per cent of people aged sixty-plus who fracture their hip will lose the ability to wash themselves, dress themselves or walk across a room unaided.
- 90 per cent of hip fractures are due to osteoporosis.

In post-menopause, the IOS recommends an annual DXA scan because significant bone loss occurs post-menopause for approximately ten years. Since bone loss is silent, repeat scanning is the only way to determine if a sudden decline is occurring.

The IOS also recommends an annual DXA scan if your initial results are positive for bone loss, as you have been diagnosed with a disease and therefore it should be monitored. Any decline in your DXA scan results should be investigated. The horse has bolted once you suffer a fracture, so this is one aspect of your health I would strongly encourage you to be proactive with.

If you have a DXA scan eleven years post-menopause and it is negative, the IOS recommends that you wait five years for a repeat DXA scan, as long as you have no current risk factors for bone loss, and do not develop a condition or are put on a medication or treatment that can cause bone loss.

FURTHER TESTS

There is a significant number of blood tests that should be done if a person has bone loss: vitamin D, parathyroid hormone (PTH), calcium, kidney function, PINP (a sensitive marker of bone formation), CTX1 (a marker for osteoporosis and bone reabsorption) and osteocalcin, to name a few. Calcium levels on their own are not sufficient.

CONDITIONS LINKED TO BONE HEALTH

Coeliac disease

This disease often comes on in menopause and it can be common for coeliacs to have bone-health issues, which is why anyone diagnosed should have a DXA scan done: prior to the diagnosis, they may not have been absorbing nutrients such as calcium, vitamin D and protein, which are essential to bone health. A large study reported a higher incidence of fractures in coeliac sufferers compared to non-sufferers, with increases of 90 per cent and almost 80 per cent for hip and wrist fractures respectively.

If diagnosed early enough and if a gluten-free diet is followed, long-term bone health is likely to be unaffected.

Sarcopenia

Maybe you had strong, lean muscles before perimenopause kicked in and now gradually that's all changing. You're no longer so lean and toned. Lower levels of oestrogen and declining testosterone impact our muscles. Sarcopenia refers to a progressive and generalised loss of muscle mass and strength due to ageing. After thirty, muscle mass decreases by about 3 to 8 per cent per decade, and after sixty, the rate of decline is higher. So as we think about building our bone health, we also need to factor in strengthening our muscles: healthy muscle equals healthy bone. Impact, strengthening and resistance all work your bones and muscles, and it is essential now that we challenge our bodies outside their comfort zone.

I firmly believe a multifactorial, proactive approach to our health is essential. Yes, we may need to advocate for our own health needs more strongly than our male counterparts, but as well as going down the medical route, there are many lifestyle factors we can address too – strength training as well as Pilates, improving balance to reduce risks of falls, looking at our nutrition, reducing alcohol intake and finding ways to reduce chronic stress. In my personal experience, this approach has worked and my T scores have improved over time.

– Steph

MAINTAINING BONE HEALTH

The impact of stress on your bones

Our bones are stimulated not just by movement and activity. They are also impacted by our stress response. Researchers at Columbia University have revealed that the osteocalcin protein, which is released by bone cells, plays a part in the fight-or-flight response. Studies of war survivors and PTSD victims all showed a higher risk of developing osteoporosis due to the psychological stress they had experienced.

Stress also impacts your behaviour, so your sleep, eating and exercise habits will change, which can have a negative effect on your bone health. The shock of a diagnosis of osteoporosis can result in anxiety and loss of social interaction, both of which further exacerbate stress. In my experience, there appears to be a stigma with this diagnosis, similar to how depression was considered ten years ago. It is important that we openly discuss osteoporosis, as we are now doing with menopause. Managing your stress has a positive impact on bone health and much more.

Movement

This is your top priority for bone and muscle health. Your focus should be on weight-bearing exercise – activities that put weight on your joints and bones – and resistance training, alongside all other forms of exercise you may be doing. Strength and balance are pivotal.

Here are some tips for exercising:

- Progressive resistance training (lifting weights) and high-impact exercise (for example, jumping or rope skipping) increase bone mineral density by 1 to 4 per cent per year in pre- and post-menopausal women.

- Weight-bearing aerobic exercise of moderate to high intensity, such as running, dancing, basketball or tennis would be an ideal addition to your regime. More vigorous exercise produces greater effects.

- One large study showed a benefit from brisk walking in reducing the risk of hip fracture (more than four hours a week may reduce the risk by 41 per cent). However, the pace needs to be altered periodically, for example every five minutes, rather than maintaining the same speed, since bone responds better to different strains, and the route needs to be altered for the most benefit.

- Short bursts of high-intensity and/or high-impact activities such as jogging, jumping, running, dancing and rope skipping are more stimulating to bone cells than sustained low-impact activities, such as walking, and also excellent for the health of your muscles.

- In resistance training, lifting heavy weights is more effective than lifting light weights (be sure to build up your strength gradually to avoid injury).

- Power training, where you lift heavy weights faster, seems to be more effective than lifting heavy weights slowly.

- Non-weight-bearing aerobic activity (such as swimming or cycling) does not improve bone density.

- Fast movements are more stimulating than slow movements.

- Check out specific exercises for muscles connected to the key bones prone to fracture – hip, wrist and mid-spine.

- Ideally, aim for 150 minutes per week of moderate to intense exercise *and* two resistance sessions.

Caveat: A person can look perfectly fine on the outside but have severe bone loss. If you have osteopenia and/or osteoporosis, you should consult a chartered physiotherapist who regularly treats those with bone loss. Everyone should be individually assessed for a safe and appropriate exercise programme. What stretches, exercises and activities are safe for you should be based on your risk of bone loss, history of broken bones, DXA results and your medical history.

Menu

Pay attention to the nutrient robbers (see Chapter 19) – reducing your intake of caffeine, alcohol and soft drinks is a must. Caffeine is in tea, coffee, energy and some soft drinks, and it can cause us to excrete calcium in our urine. Energy and soft drinks also contain phosphorus, which may deplete calcium in the bones.

Protein provides the essential amino acids that support bone building and healthy muscles. Studies show that a low protein diet is linked to loss of bone mineral density in older people. Make a point to incorporate it into every meal or snack and especially into your breakfast.

Calcium

This mineral is very important for bone health, but it's not the only factor. Calcium makes your bones stronger and improves bone quality and is also needed for healthy nerves and muscle function. It is a major building block of your body. Calcium requirements peak at two life stages: during adolescence (rapid growth) and for people over fifty (ability to absorb calcium starts to decline). Our bones store calcium, so if there is not enough in the body for daily use, it will take what it needs from the bones. This is not a good thing, as it weakens the bones.

Calcium through your food is the first port of call. Good sources include milk and dairy products; green vegetables such as broccoli, curly kale and bok choy; whole canned fish with soft, edible bones such as sardines; nuts (almonds and Brazil nuts are mighty); and calcium-set tofu. The recommended dietary intake is 1,300mg per day.

If you do not get enough through your diet, a supplement is a good idea, and the World Health Organisation recommends no higher than 500–600mg per day. This should be combined with vitamin D and vitamin K for absorption.

Vitamin D

Sun exposure with SPF will support vitamin D production, which helps calcium absorption in the body. This vitamin plays an essential role in bone and muscle development. It can contribute to reducing fracture risk by regulating calcium levels in the body and helping absorb calcium from the intestine, improving muscle performance and balance – thus reducing fall risks. Vitamin D deficiency in adults can result in osteomalacia, which is a softening of the bones due to poor mineralisation.

Magnesium

A critical ingredient in bone health, magnesium protects our bones, muscles and blood vessels. It is often forgotten about when it comes to bone health. (See Chapter 16 for more.)

Silicon

A deficiency in silicon leads to poor skeletal development, as it plays an essential role in bone formation. Sources include whole grains, carrots and green beans.

Vitamin K

Low vitamin K impacts bone health and strength. Vitamins K1 and K2 are the ones you may have heard of, but it is K2 that improves bone density – it directs calcium into the bones and keeps it out of the soft tissues (arteries). Sources of K2 are fermented foods and grass-fed protein.

Boron

Because boron is a trace element, your body doesn't require vast amounts of it. However, it's important, as it makes calcium absorption possible. Additionally, boron can help trigger the vitamins and minerals required for strong bone growth. It acts positively on calcium, phosphorus, magnesium and vitamin D. It is an often-forgotten element of bone health. Prunes, avocados, raisins, peaches, peanuts, apples and broccoli are good sources of boron.

HRT

Oestrogen has a protective effect on your bones and is used to promote bone health. It has a key role in maintaining bone and preventing bone loss. (See Chapter 14.) HRT can be an effective treatment where both osteoporosis and menopause symptoms exist.

KEEPING YOURSELF SAFE

Menopause offers us a window of opportunity to prepare for our future health. It's never too early to start considering practical ways to support your bones:

- Install easy-grip handrails, particularly on stairs
- Don't use wax on the floor and remove all loose rugs
- Install bars for getting in and out of the bath or shower (grab bars are easy to find and don't need screws)
- Ensure good lighting
- If possible, avoid long clothes that you could trip on
- Have regular eye checks
- Reduce the need for bending and climbing – adjust the height of items where needed

* * *

You can protect your bone health through exercise, the right foods, reducing nutrient robbers and making lifestyle changes that support you in these years. Don't forget: the steps here will enhance your muscle health as well, and this too is crucial. Start now, however small – even with just a brisk ten-minute walk. Incorporate movement into your daily life, and your bountiful bones will thank you!

8

Maintaining a healthy brain

What have you forgotten over the last few days? Has it been at work? Brain fog, fuzzy brain, the word on the tip of your tongue that just disappears, leaving you feeling disjointed, scattered, unfocused and scared? Has a to-do list become essential?

This is not Alzheimer's. This is one of the most common symptoms of menopause and post-menopause as our bodies adapt to the changing and finally lower levels of oestrogen in the brain. A huge number of women suffer from a variety of psychological symptoms during perimenopause and menopause, including anxiety, panic attacks, brain fog and feelings of invisibility.

Brain fog is one symptom that has given me, personally, considerable hassle, especially in the early perimenopause years. I was working full time, had three kids and a busy life – the perfect storm. And whatever about mishaps at home, when they happened at work it added another layer of confusion and complexity. Then add to this the very personal aspect of this chapter: a family history of dementia. This is a cruel disease – those of you who have known someone with it will understand all too well. It is a disease we all want to do our utmost to avoid, a stark reminder of the importance of future-proofing our cognitive function.

YOUR FABULOUS BRAIN

In traditional Chinese medicine, menopause and the accompanying age has been revered by society – a woman is seen as being at her pinnacle of wisdom and a source of vital support for her community. In the West, the narrative is different. During perimenopause, the average woman is chasing after children, caring for ageing parents, holding down a job, rushing back to get dinner and look after the house. In today's world, you may be working from home, where the boundaries have become murky and work life slips easily into home life – another added stress. It's extreme multitasking – our poor brains! Women carry heavy mental loads, and when this is constant our brains need support.

Brain fog is one of the heavy hitters in perimenopause. You go to the cupboard and haven't a clue what you were looking for; you're talking to someone familiar and completely forget their name. It is common and it is, unfortunately, all part of the process – as we get older, our circulation slows down, so less oxygen is circulated around the body and the brain. Also, as oestrogen stimulates the neurotransmitters in the brain, the changing hormone levels that come at midlife slow these down, so our brains aren't working at peak performance. The end result is that our brain isn't as sharp as it was in our twenties. Many women report fear of dementia, fear of losing their mind – and it can certainly feel like that. The good news is that there are many ways to improve our brain function and eliminate the brain fog and cloudiness.

BRAIN POWER

Your brain is the master conductor, the control room of your body. It's always working, even as you sleep, sending and receiving essential messages throughout your body. Everything you experience in your day goes via your brain. If a spider lands on you, a message fires to the brain. You either brush it off or jump. These messages travel faster than any bullet train. Neurotransmitters are the chemical messengers that transport these messages from one neuron to the next until they reach their destination. Here are some of the key ones:

- Serotonin (aka the happy hormone) is responsible for signals related to sleep, body temperature, mood and pain.
- Dopamine is key for movement and posture (low levels are a factor in the muscle rigidity that impacts Parkinson's disease). This can also be linked to addictive-type behaviour.
- Noradrenaline is similar to adrenaline, which is involved in the fight-or-flight response. It keeps us alert and focused.
- Acetylcholine plays a role in attention, wakefulness, learning and memory. Very low levels are found in people with dementia.

These are just some of the many neurotransmitters working away in your brain even now as you read these lines. All of them have an impact on your life at every stage.

HORMONES AND YOUR BRAIN

By now you understand the wide-reaching impact of the key hormones of oestrogen, progesterone and testosterone on the body. They also have a huge influence on the brain.

The effects of oestrogen on your brain function are immense – as oestrogen levels change, it has a ripple effect on all aspects of life. Mood swings, depression and sleep issues all impact and heighten brain fog. Oestrogen gives our brains that spark, making us alert and efficient.

Thinking of oestrogen as 'fuel for the brain', as Dr Lisa Mosconi refers to it, makes so much sense when we look at its far-reaching implications. In Alzheimer's and dementia, we hear about a protein called beta-amyloid that accumulates in the brain. Oestrogen offers a protection against this build-up, and changes in oestrogen levels also have a knock-on impact on the neurotransmitters mentioned earlier and, in particular, how we process serotonin, which then impacts cognition. Variable amounts of oestrogen can also affect blood flow, which may contribute to migraine symptoms. (For more in-depth information on brain health, I would urge you to read Dr Mosconi's *The XX Brain*.)

While we think of the ovaries as the centre point for the symptoms and activities related to menopause, we now know menopause impacts the brain too. Remember those messengers and relationships we talked about earlier? They all start in the brain, the master conductor.

Progesterone, on the other hand, works in a kind of opposing way to oestrogen and calms the brain down. It can make you feel drowsy and it helps reduce anxiety.

Throughout your life these two hormones work in tandem. Our menstrual cycles are reliant on the peak in oestrogen in the first part to peaking progesterone in the latter part. So in perimenopause, as the body adapts to hormonal changes, the partnership between these two hormones can go out of balance. All this activity stems from the brain and the intricate network of connections between the pituitary gland and the hypothalamus, the master regulator in the stimulation of oestrogen and progesterone production in the ovaries.

Testosterone also has a role to play with the receptors in the brain. A Polish study of post-menopausal women with high or normal levels of DHEA (a precursor of testosterone) showed they experienced better cognitive function and memory.

WHAT ABOUT AGEING?

Ageing and hormonal changes collide when it comes to our lovely brains. I want you to make your brain your best friend from here on. Appreciate it, and be grateful for all it does. It wakes you up; it signals to your body to move throughout the day; it influences your mood, how sharp and on the ball you are on any given day; it is the part of you that gives you your voice and helps you speak. It protects you. It can calm you. It is miraculous on a daily basis.

And we need to embrace ageing too. Like menopause, it is inevitable, and that means some parts of our brains will shrink, with the cognitive aspects generally being the first to be impacted. The all-important blood flow inside the brain and going to the brain starts to slow down. Inflammation may also start to increase in your brain and other parts of your body. This is why taking steps now to protect your cognitive function are crucial. I know you may already be overwhelmed with symptoms of menopause, but I would urge you to use these years to build optimum health for the future.

DEMENTIA AND ALZHEIMER'S

Two out of three dementia and Alzheimer's patients are women. Unfortunately, we are more prone than men to these conditions. They don't just come on overnight – they commence many years before diagnosis, showing no symptoms whatsoever. Current research indicates that they start in the menopause years, and possibly before, and are also impacted by genetic, lifestyle and medical factors.

If you think of coronary heart disease as a heart illness, then Alzheimer's is a disease of the brain. Symptoms may arise twenty years before you actually notice – subtle changes start in the brain but don't interfere with your daily life, so you are not aware. Those nerve cells in your brain (neurons) that perform the roles of thinking, memory and learning are damaged or destroyed. Over time, this extends to other parts of the brain outside the key cognitive areas.

Dementia is an overarching term referring to a set of symptoms. The hallmarks of dementia are issues with memory, language, learning, problem-solving and everyday thinking skills that can affect a person's life. Alzheimer's is the most common form of dementia; 60–80 per cent of dementia cases are Alzheimer's.

Risks for Alzheimer's

Here are some common risk factors for Alzheimer's:

- Genetics: if a parent has had this disease, you will have a susceptibility or predisposition also. It is not a given, but a risk, so ensuring you take preventative steps is crucial. Here too you may come across the APOE gene. We all have these genes but there are variants, 2, 3 and 4, all of which have a different impact on your health. APOE-4 is the gene linked to Alzheimer's.
- Ethnicity also has a part to play, with US studies showing that African American women are twice as likely to develop this disease.
- Medical issues like heart disease, diabetes, obesity, thyroid, brain injury, inflammation, infections and depression also add to risk.
- Environment and lifestyle play a huge part here too. Maintaining a healthy diet and managing stress are the foundations of future-proofing your brain health.

Thyroid disease

The symptoms of a thyroid imbalance can look very similar to those of menopause. They can also mirror the symptoms of dementia, which is why keeping an eye on your thyroid health should be part of your ongoing maintenance and habits.

WHAT IS BRAIN FOG?

Brain fog is real – any hormonal woman (whether due to monthly cycles, pregnancy or menopause) can attest to this fact. It has been defined as 'forgetfulness, difficulty concentrating and thinking clearly'. The collision of hormonal changes and other key brain hormones like serotonin create it. The SWAN study, which encompassed over three thousand women, found that brain fog is due to low oestrogen levels, which impact the hippocampus (a key part of the brain that looks after memory), and also noted that brain fog is heightened when you are feeling stressed, exhausted and overwhelmed. Think of a typical night in menopause where you are sleep deprived due to worry or night sweats – your brain fog is always worse the next day. Those key neurotransmitters aren't firing as they should; they are touchy, tired and grouchy, so messages are not sent as they should be.

CHANGE: COGNITIVE FUNCTION'S BEST FRIEND

Our brains like to be challenged: they want to grow and expand in new directions. As you read all the ideas below to nourish your brain health, remember how important it is to bring ongoing change into the equation. If I run the same distance and same route every time, there is no challenge. Variety is key. Whether with food, exercise or lifestyle, keep adding to the mix and incorporating changes along the way. And on the flip side, try to fit your regular tasks into an existing routine, leaving you with more time for your creative side – do some stretches while the kettle boils, build ten minutes' meditation into your night-time wind-down. Our brains hover between change and routine, with both being beneficial.

TIPS TO ACHIEVE OPTIMAL BRAIN FUNCTION
Neuro-nutrition

A new area of research is emerging called neuro-nutrition, which reinforces the importance of taking care of our brain health. This approach looks at the body as a whole and not just the brain. The gut–brain connection has been understood for a number of years now: how our daily nutrition impacts our brains, at all life stages. With healthy lifestyle choices, reduced stress and nutritional support, we can help our brains both heal and regenerate.

The Mediterranean diet and omega-3 fatty acids: About 60 per cent of your brain is composed of fat, so essential fatty acids (EFAs) are important. Our bodies cannot make them so we must include them in our diets. These EFAs include omega-3, -6 and -9, with omega-3 being the most important due to its anti-inflammatory properties. The Mediterranean diet, with its focus on olive oil, fruits, vegetables and wholegrains, consists of many foods rich in omega-3 and offers great support in maintaining optimal brain function. Omega-3 is the only fat that consistently goes into the brain, where it's used to build brain and nerve cells. The Mediterranean diet is also linked to lowering bad cholesterol and promoting heart health. Extra virgin olive oil is a big part of this – be diligent when buying your oil, as not all bottles are the same quality. Watch for its origin, the date bottled and that it's not a blend of olives (ideally, they should be from one country).

Antioxidants: These are crucial: they travel around your body sweeping up harmful free radicals, which can cause cell damage and disease. Blackberries (which are higher in vitamin C than blueberries), apples, sweet potatoes, parsnips, brown rice and buckwheat are all good sources of antioxidants.

Gut health: Almost a second brain, the gut communicates regularly with our brain, affecting our moods and energy levels. Probiotics provide significant antioxidant protection and lessen the risk of developing a number of inflammation-based conditions that can affect the brain. Fermented foods are great sources of probiotics. (See Chapter 19 for more.)

Water, water, water!

Having spoken to thousands of women, I can safely say that few of us drink enough water. In menopause, it becomes a double-edged sword because if you are experiencing urinary issues you will feel like reducing your fluid intake. Please don't. It's essential. Your brain is 80 per cent water – this is reason enough to consume water on a regular basis.

Dehydration is no friend to the brain or to perimenopause. It has a huge impact on anxiety and brain fog. Water is essential for optimal brain function: it prevents dehydration and increases the blood's circulation – both of which stave off cognitive decline and nerve damage.

And it's not just your brain: your heart is 73 per cent water, the lungs over 80 per cent. Water is essential for metabolism, so sufficient intake is essential in weight management.

Ensure you drink a minimum of eight glasses of room-temperature water a day – ideally good mineral or spring water via a filtration system. The minerals in water are almost as essential as the water itself – coconut water is a powerful rehydration tool because of its minerals and electrolytes. Drinking warm water in the morning promotes metabolism and gives your body a good kick-start – try it with some fresh ginger or lemon. (Don't forget: certain foods also contain lots of water – for more, see Chapter 19.)

Avoid alcohol

Too much alcohol has a definite impact on our brain functioning, and if you do experience 'foggy brain' then I would suggest staying away from it. Even one glass a day will impact you if you are already experiencing symptoms of brain fog.

Polyphenols

There *is* good news, especially if you are a red-wine drinker. Chocolate and red wine contain polyphenols, which are antioxidants. Red wine contains resveratrol, a very-good-to-have antioxidant – excellent at reducing inflammation in your body.

The best sources of polyphenols are berries, dark chocolate, coffee, spices like cloves and star anise and the odd glass of red wine.

Diets and blood sugar levels

Our bodies need glucose (which is an energy source) to function: this is what lies behind a balanced blood sugar level. Your brain uses half of all the glucose produced in your body – according to Harvard Medical School it is the 'most energy-demanding organ'. And this leads us to diets. Personally, I am not a fan of diets – I am more for establishing a healthy way of eating throughout your life. I have spoken with women who are 'dieting' and really struggling in menopause, as the diet they are following may restrict times when they can eat. Starving yourself during the day will not help you in menopause. Your memory and concentration may suffer as a result, and brain fog may increase.

Alzheimer's has recently been referred to by some scientists as type 3 diabetes, or diabetes of the brain (though it's a controversial term). This is because scientists have found how important insulin is to the brain. Ongoing research is happening in this area and may lead to further understanding of whether dementia might also be impacted by metabolic changes.

Supplements

Magnesium and B vitamins are really important for the brain, with the emphasis on vitamins B6, B9, B12 and choline. Our nervous system and ageing blood vessels benefit from these nutrients.

L-carnitine is an amino acid derivative found in red meat. It is easily absorbed by the body and the brain and may improve neurotransmitter activity, mitochondrial function and cognition.

Vitamin E's benefit comes from its antioxidant properties. While it has been used in several clinical trials for Alzheimer's, its benefit as a preventative for neurodegenerative disease is not known, but it may help improve your memory and concentration. However, if you are on blood pressure medication, please check with your doctor before starting vitamin E.

Limited research has been done into vitamin A's impact on brain health, but studies to date indicate that this vitamin has an important role to play in the health of your brain.

Vitamin C has wide-ranging benefits for the brain. As we age, our brains generate fewer neurotransmitters, such as the key ones mentioned earlier – dopamine, acetylcholine, serotonin and norepinephrine (also known as noradrenaline). This decrease in their activity may play a role in declining cognition and memory. Vitamin C helps your brain cells to effectively use these important neurological chemicals, playing a role in influencing cognitive performance. Vitamin C is also a powerful antioxidant. Research has shown that higher levels of free radicals, the by-products of oxidation (the process by which we make energy in our cells), are associated with age-related cognitive impairment. Studies have shown that vitamin C can reduce the potential effects of these oxidative products on cognitive function.

Vitamin D, often a very underrated vitamin, is key to bone health, immunity, calcium absorption and neurodevelopment.

If you don't get enough omega-3 in your diet, it is worth looking at a good supplement, as this is one of the most important nutrients in perimenopause.

Herbal medicine

Can herbs help our brains? The answer, I believe, is yes. I have used herbal tonics for many years and believe they can play a powerful role – in particular *Ginkgo biloba*, ashwagandha and turmeric, as well as lion's mane and reishi mushrooms.

Physical exercise

Exercise has been promoted as a possible preventative measure against neurodegenerative disease – this includes both physical and brain exercise. Aerobic exercise has been linked to a significant increase in brain volume and cognitive function in midlife. It is also believed that exercise has an anti-inflammatory effect that promotes brain health.

Exercise intensity is all important here:

- Easy/light: this will increase brain volume and reduce risk of cognitive decline. You are aiming here for a heart rate of 114–132 bpm, or beats per minute. (We all differ when it comes to heart rate – yours may be lower or higher than average, so it is best to become familiar with your bpm.)
- Getting focused/moderate: here you are keeping your brain young; memory, cognitive functioning and mood are improved. Aim for 133–151 bpm.

- Pumping it/hard: now you're getting serious – you're building new brain cells and ticking all the previous boxes. Aim for 152–170 bpm.
- Elite style/maximum heart rate: now you're into elite brain health – you are boosting a key protein that helps grow new brain cells and ticks all the previous boxes.

Aim to exercise for thirty minutes five times per week where you get to the stage of feeling breathless. This gives an oxygen boost to the body and releases feel-good hormones. This can be 150 minutes of moderate activity or 75 minutes of hard or maximum activity a week.

What is most important is picking an exercise that you like – this is a life habit, and you'll find it easier to establish if you enjoy it. Consider any exercise, and if it can also promote bone and muscle health (see Chapter 7) then you're achieving two things with one action.

Mental exercise

With on average 70,000 thoughts per day, our minds need respite. Exercise for the brain can be anything that challenges you mentally – for example, learning a new language or craft, doing puzzles, using your non-dominant hand to colour or write for a few minutes each day or reading a book outside your normal reading list. You could also try some brain-training apps – there are lots to choose from.

Meditation and mindfulness are very helpful brain exercises that I would also encourage you to investigate.

The power of music

Learning a new musical instrument offers great benefits to our brains – you could even take up an instrument you played as a child but have put aside for many years. It's like learning a new language: you are challenging your brain to learn something new and think in a new way, and this is excellent for creating and enhancing neural pathways.

But don't worry if you don't have the talent of Mozart or Chopin – you can still benefit from listening to music that you like. It's another form of giving your brain exercise and an easy and nice addition to your daily habits. So get that Spotify playlist going or delve back into your old records or CDs and rekindle your love of music.

My daughter wanted to give up piano last year – I took a vagary and asked her teacher if I could take the lessons instead. I've always loved music and I played piano for a few years as a kid, but I didn't enjoy it – I wasn't interested in classical music and felt oppressed by having to practise. Now it's a completely different experience! I have the confidence to ask questions and say what I want to explore. I'm learning how music works and figuring out how to play what I love. There's no pressure, but at the same time, I've made a commitment to myself to practise every day. It's the most joyful time – the sense of achievement when I finally get something I've been struggling with, the excitement of learning, of just doing something different, outside of work and family, for myself alone. Sometimes I'll lift my head to find I've been there for an hour when I only meant to spend fifteen minutes!

– Emma

Relaxation and stress management

Multitasking is no friend of menopause: make a change to single-tasking. You probably have a lot going on in your life already on a daily basis, and finding time to stop and rest can be an added pressure on top of an endless to-do list. But it's *crucial*. I have spoken with many women who have really felt the pressure of brain fog in their workday, from lawyers to busy mums running from one after-school activity to the next, from retail assistants to nurses. It impacts us all on some level.

A busy life equals a busy brain. Remember all those vital jobs our wonderful brain does for us? We need to give it a rest, some respite from the endless chatter.

Look at the daily stressors in your life and try to find ways you can eliminate or reduce them: the less stress in your life, the greater your ability to focus and pay attention. Also consider some form of daily relaxation like mindfulness or meditation that gives your brain a complete rest from the busyness of life (see Chapter 18).

Sleep

Chapter 4 delves into this in more detail, but I always say 'Sleep is the bedrock of thriving through menopause'. None of us functions at our optimum when we have missed a few hours of good deep sleep. Our brain needs this down time to process the day's events and renew itself. It's a time for rest, a time for healing and restoring your immune system. Sleep is the cheapest form of therapy you can get, with your hippocampus working away to clear out unwanted information from your day. If you are feeling exhausted, your serotonin levels will drop and that impacts melatonin, the trigger to put us asleep. If our sleep is not deep and restorative, that free overnight therapy that operates when our eyes are closed will not work effectively. When you have had a night of hot flushes or night sweats, you will automatically feel more tired the following day – both in your body and your brain.

Review your sleep habits and consider making small tweaks to ensure you are getting your required amount of sleep per night – for some people it's six hours, for others eight.

Reduce screen time

From Netflix to smartphones, our lives are now centred around screens and our brains are always looking for those notifications and alerts. Many of us also spend long portions of the day at work using screens, so a rest from them is essential. Some tips for reducing screen time are to put time limits on social media apps and turn off notifications. Using night mode on your mobile device could help with eye strain.

Socialise

Staying connected with others is a key element for thriving through menopause. Menopause can be lonely. Being with people is imperative to keep your brain nourished. Neuroplasticity shows us how the brain is continually changing, and social interactions are a key part of this. (See Chapter 20.)

Mind your hearing

Our hearing will naturally reduce over the coming years, so doing what you can to protect it is a must. Deafness increases your risk of dementia – the direct link isn't yet known but possibly it's the impact it may have on social interaction. To protect your hearing as best you can:

- Have your hearing monitored by an audiologist so you have a benchmark for the coming years – have it reviewed every five years.
- Avoid loud environments. Wear earplugs while mowing the lawn (better yet, leave that one to someone else!), on a plane or at concerts. Take a break, too, every so often from the noise. It takes on average eighteen hours for your ears to resettle after a loud concert.
- Watch research about headphones – it seems to be moving fast here in relation to the downsides of using earbuds. If using them, take a five-minute break every hour. Don't have them on maximum volume – aim for 60 per cent or less.

Chew gum

I came across the power of chewing gum when I was researching anxiety a few years ago and discovered that it can help your mood. A 2015 study showed that chewing gum can result in enhanced productivity and fewer cognitive errors at work. And you don't need to chew like a rabbit – the rate of chewing did not impact the results.

Look after your teeth

Thousands of different bacteria live in your mouth – good and bad. This bacteria forms a thin film on your teeth called plaque. If it builds up and hardens, your gums can become inflamed. Over time, if left untreated, it can lead to gum disease, or gingivitis. But it doesn't stop in your mouth. It can move past the gums into your immune system, invading the white blood cells. This particular strain of bacteria can even reach your brain. A 2019 study on the brains of people who died from dementia found that the majority contained *Porphyromonas gingivalis*, the main bacteria involved in gum disease.

How to look after your teeth:

- See your dentist regularly. Sore gums, bleeding and bad breath are all signs of gingivitis.
- Brush twice a day and floss. Floss breaks up the plaque that builds up between your teeth.
- Use a soft brush – don't go too hard on your teeth or gums.
- Tartar is plaque build-up – you will need your dentist or hygienist to remove it.
- Quit smoking.

HRT AND BRAIN HEALTH

Studies have been done, and there is anecdotal information from women, but at the time of writing there is no published research on whether HRT will prevent dementia. As mentioned earlier, this is a rapidly evolving area. Research undertaken by neuroscientists such as Dr Lisa Mosconi have demonstrated changes in the structure of the brain during the menopause transition that is separate to and different from that of chronological ageing. It is hypothesised that starting HRT for genetically vulnerable individuals might negate or reduce this risk – but more data is needed to be able to analyse this in more detail.

What we do know, according to the International Menopause Society and the British Menopause Society:

- HRT is of no help if you have a diagnosis of dementia.
- HRT should not be given for the prevention or treatment of cognitive difficulties.

And what about the specific type of oestrogen the brain itself produces – neuroestradiol? A study from 2013 showed its importance as a neuro-transmitter. Unlike the oestrogen in the body, though, we cannot yet measure the oestrogen in the brain.

Making an informed decision with any form of medication is key. Many women say they feel brain function improves with oestrogen alone and that at the times of their HRT regime when they are taking progesterone they may not feel the same clarity.

DOES IT GET BETTER AFTER MENOPAUSE?

This is the million-dollar question. We need to factor two things in here: ageing and the transition that is menopause.

Ageing will bring changes to memory and cognitive function, and we know that for many women the menopause years are, in fact, as Dr Lisa Mosconi calls it, a recalibration of the brain – a resetting. Your brain is working from a different place after menopause: you are different; so too is your brain. You are still you – it may just be that you are not accessing information as quickly as you did before. This recalibration, for the majority of women, will settle down after menopause, with the common symptoms of brain fog fading into the background. And when those moments strike, remember that if you pause, take a breath and calmly ask your brain to recall and revisit events, it will probably do it. Take a breather, step away and gently let things come back to you.

Accepting the new level that your brain is now working at and being kind and gentle to yourself will make a world of difference. And what can we gain from a calmer brain, the move away from the never-ending thoughts that besiege us? Your brain is changing as you read this – why not accept that for the inevitable transition it is and take those crucial lifestyle steps and treatment options that will support your brain, not just for these years but to ensure optimum brain health when you are in your seventies, eighties and nineties.

Looking after your body in menopause is not just about symptom management, it is about future-proofing your health, and your cognitive health is one of the most important aspects. Take it from the daughter of a strong, successful businesswoman who would have hated to end her days with dementia.

9

When things get hot – the vasomotor symptoms

Feeling like a volcano is sweeping over you, a hot wave full of intense heat – heat that leaves you quaking in your boots with the speed at which it overtakes your body? Drenched clothes and face that make you want to jump into the nearest body of water, regardless of the fact that it's winter?

Who doesn't associate hot flushes with menopause, the stereotypical symptom that can cause intense disruption to your life? Hot flushes and night sweats are referred to as vasomotor symptoms and will be different for each woman. Around 75 per cent of all women experience these rapid, short and recurring rises in body temperature, peaking in the late perimenopause years. Hot flushes usually begin before a woman's last period and last two years or less for 80 per cent of women. For many, they can continue into the post-menopause years and generally are the last symptom that you may experience.

If you are going through any of the forms of early menopause, and bypassing perimenopause itself, the chances are you may feel these symptoms more intensely than others. Surgical menopause will often see women experience intense hot flushes and night sweats within days of surgery.

The flushes came relentlessly, wave after wave, and wearing warm clothing even in winter became impossible unless I could get it off really quickly. Then the cold sweats at the end and a clammy feeling, so from red hot to clammy cold, one spectrum to another. Sleeping became a nightmare of insomnia or sheets on/sheets off all night, so much less sleep. I even lay on the bathroom floor on cold tiles to get cool at one point, as the heat was too much to bear.

Dealing with these symptoms meant using fans, cold water, visualising freezers, physically going into supermarkets to open the freezer doors and stand in them to get cold quick, taking clothing off rapidly – the sensation of heat brought panic, anxiety and a need to just get cold fast. Plus the overwhelming desire to strip off just to get cold quickly! My confidence started to ebb away. I knew when they were coming and started to lose eye contact and finish talking quickly so I could move away from people before I went deep red and got wet through. It affected my life, my confidence and my ability to do my job.

– Liz

WHAT IS A HOT FLUSH?

You may also hear it referred to as a hot flash or a power surge – whatever you call it, once you experience one you will know. This isn't a soft wave of warmth covering you: this is an intense flame of fire that quickly spreads through the arms, chest, neck and face. Your body will feel warm when one hits, and it can also come with skin redness, nausea, sweating and anxiety. You may feel like your heart is beating faster than normal (see Chapter 11). When a hot flush occurs at night-time and causes excess sweating in bed, that's a night sweat. Again, this will differ for all. Many will experience drenching night sweats, where they go through several sets of pyjamas in one night, while for others they may be mild enough that they sleep through them. For many women, night sweats bring soaked sheets, disturbed sleep, restless sleep and dehydration.

The worst symptoms had to be the electric goosebumps on my thighs that announced the arrival of a hot flush. It would move up into my stomach and wake me. It was horrendous.

– Noreen

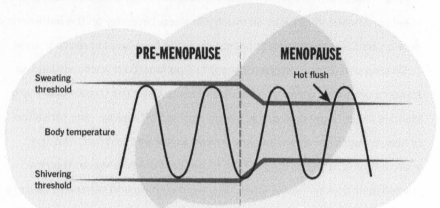

Hot flushes are all part of thermoregulation. Our body temperature goes between established thresholds that are regulated by the hypothalamus, one of the key parts of the brain. When the hypothalamus sees that our body temperature is going up or down, it kicks the body into action.

In menopause, the thermostat isn't operating as it should, so it tells your brain that you're hot when you are not. In perimenopause the established thresholds change – the hot threshold moves down, the cold moves up. You now have both a narrower thermostat and heightened sensitivity to even the smallest changes in your body temperature.

A hot flush happens when the brain experiences a change in oestrogen levels. This change results in a heightened thermoregulation system – small changes, which your body would have quietly adapted to before, now become a big issue. The signalling in the brain to the body is out of kilter. Oestrogen drops also impact the levels of serotonin and adrenaline, which will have an impact on the hypothalamus. This is why we can see a direct correlation between stress management and a reduction in the duration and frequency of hot flushes – research indicates relaxation will help reduce the occurrences of hot flushes.

The body must respond to signals from the brain, and it does so by dilating blood vessels and sending blood to the outer layer – the skin – in an effort to cool things down. This is the hot flush. Your heart rate will also go up and you may perspire profusely.

It can last from two to four minutes and you may experience twenty to thirty a day. And then ... you get cold! How unfair is that? But remember, you were never actually hot: it was your out-of-kilter thermoregulation that kicked this all off. It can create a vicious cycle of disrupted sleep and increased anxiety. For 20 per cent of women, hot flushes can be severe and cause real havoc to their quality of life.

Other factors that can make you more prone to vasomotor symptoms are smoking, ethnicity, mental health problems, anxiety, alcohol and caffeine intake.

> I then decided to deal with the lack of confidence and announced to whoever I was speaking to that, if I unfortunately went fire-engine red, please not to call for an ambulance as it's just a temporary hot moment. I found by telling people I remained calm and in control and could deal with any heated moments, and most times I did not get any flushes after saying it out loud.
>
> – Liz

What about cold flushes?

Yes, they can happen! A cold flush is a tingling, shivering and freezing sensation that can strike at any time. It may also cause you to tremble or become pale. A chilly flush is usually brief, lasting only a few minutes. Cold flushes are sometimes linked to menopause, although they can be triggered by other hormonal or emotional changes (thyroid imbalance being one). They can also be a symptom of cardiovascular disease in women (see Chapter 11). Cold flushes can occur, too, in people who are stressed, resulting in insomnia and even more anxious thoughts. We know that Japanese women experience cold flushes more than women in the West (stiff, frozen shoulders being another common symptom). The advice is the same, with the exception of adding layers to keep you warm and, if it's happening at night-time, wearing bed socks to help.

When can they start?

For many women, hot flushes will start well into perimenopause. Keep an eye out for night sweats building up to or during your period, as this is frequently when they begin. And remember, also, you may never experience them. At the time of writing this, I have not yet had a hot flush, just mild night sweats. But I am well aware this may change!

As for how long they can last – well, it really is a question of how long is a piece of string. The oldest woman I spoke with who was still experiencing hot flushes was seventy-seven – that's not common but it can happen (10 per cent of women experience these symptoms for more than fifteen years).

Can they occur for reasons other than menopause?

Yes, so please ensure you rule out other possible causes – another reason an annual GP check is so crucial. Certain underlying illnesses have symptoms that look like menopause. Some things that can create hot flushes and night sweats are:

- Thyroid imbalance
- Anxiety
- Diabetes
- Sleep apnoea
- Excess alcohol consumption
- Cancer
- Tuberculosis
- Side effects of medications such as antidepressants, hormone regulators and blood sugar stabilisers

HOW TO MANAGE VASOMOTOR SYMPTOMS

Generally:

- Manage stress. It's easy to say, but I know how difficult this one is. (See Chapter 12 for more advice.)

- Try to manage your weight.
- Invest in a fan.
- Using a cooling spray.
- Wear layers of cotton clothing – during the day and in bed (for more on night sweats, see Chapter 4).
- Look to your feet. Our feet help us regulate our body temperature, so cooling your feet down may help. Try placing an ice pack under your feet for an even quicker effect.
- Keep a record of when they happen and note what was happening before the hot flush. Are they happening at certain times? After certain foods? (Spicy foods and alcohol can often trigger hot flushes or night sweats.) This will help you to learn your triggers, and then you can make small changes to gain some control over them.
- Drink enough water to keep you hydrated. Dehydration is no friend of flushes or anxiety, and even mild dehydration has been shown to negatively affect mental performance, so ensure you drink water as often as you can.

At work:

- A light scarf can be very handy.
- Sit away from a direct heat source or sunlight.
- Reduce your intake of hot drinks, especially prior to or during meetings.
- Practise breathing exercises.
- Approach your manager for onsite support (see Chapter 13).

TREATMENT OPTIONS

Exercise

Exercise has a great role to play here, with resistance training being very effective, according to clinical trials. Recent findings tell us that meditation helps reduce hot flushes by relaxing the hypothalamus, and regular exercise improves your thermoregulation.

Cognitive behavioural therapy (CBT)

What I love about CBT is its practical application. Significant research has been done into the positive impact CBT can have on the vasomotor symptoms of menopause. It works on the basis of understanding the triggers and process of what happens when you experience a hot flush or night sweats. (See also Chapter 15.)

- Physical symptoms – the hot flush or night sweat – trigger thoughts.
- Thoughts – 'Oh god, everyone can see I'm drenched'; 'Everyone can see drips of sweat on my forehead' – cause feelings.
- Feelings – anxiety, shame, embarrassment, lack of control – lead to behaviour.
- Behaviour – you may start to avoid, or become overanxious in, certain situations.

CBT asks you to look at the links between these four areas and work on a calmer, more supportive attitude to the situation:

- Physical symptoms – the hot flush or night sweat.
- Thoughts – 'This will pass'; 'Let's see how this one goes'; 'I am safe'; 'This will only last two minutes' (you can even set a timer if it helps).
- Feelings – calmer, relaxed.
- Behaviour – breathing calmly.

If possible, don't leave the situation, as this may lead to avoidance in the future and can result in social anxiety, where you may avoid people due to past experiences.

HRT

The vasomotor symptoms are generally the first to improve for many women when starting HRT. If you are using progesterone alone, like the Mirena coil, it may provide support for this symptom. (See Chapter 14 for further discussion on HRT.)

Non-hormonal medication

This can have a place where HRT is contraindicated or is not effective. Antidepressants operate by lowering adrenaline and instilling calm. Just ensure they are warranted and that other routes have been investigated. Anti-seizure medication can also be discussed with your doctor.

Acupuncture

A 2016 study showed improvements in hot-flush occurrence, sleep quality, physical symptoms, memory problems and anxiety, as well as a significant reduction in vasomotor symptoms – as much as 36.7 per cent – after a course of acupuncture. All of these advantages were maintained for at least six months after the acupuncture therapy was finished. Researchers also observed significant improvements after just three acupuncture sessions; peak clinical results were reached after an average of eight sessions.

Supplements

Magnesium, evening primrose oil, sage and maca may help – see Chapter 16 for details.

* * *

Menopause is much more than hot flushes and night sweats, but when they strike, it can certainly feel like that's all there is: a raging fire that consumes your body. But they tend to respond well to the many treatments outlined above – just find what works best for you and, as always, tackle it one symptom at a time.

10

Weight gain – what's really happening?

Weight gain can be one of the most emotive and triggering menopause symptoms. When you factor in the effects of stress, hormones, thyroid imbalance, sedentary lifestyle and pelvic floor disorders, it's easy to see why weight gain is an issue for many of us.

On average, women gain 1.5–3kg per year in these years. This may not sound like much, but over time it adds up, and it's weight that is much harder to shed – the reasons are numerous and not only menopause related but age related too.

WHAT IS HAPPENING IN YOUR BODY

Ageing, hormonal changes, body-fat composition and decreasing metabolic rate are leading causes of weight gain. In our forties and fifties, weight is harder to shift than it was in earlier years. Visceral fat now accumulates around the middle, where your organs are (before menopause, fat is generally stored around the bum and thighs). In your twenties, you might have tried the infamous cabbage soup diet or another fad diet to get into a dress and, presto, a week later all was resolved! This doesn't work in later years.

The body's metabolic rate changes, and we aren't processing food as quickly as we used to: it's on a slow burner. That lean body mass of your twenties and thirties decreases as you age. This is because of hormone changes and lifestyle changes – sitting more, commuting, less daily movement and so on. Losing this muscle mass causes us to burn fewer calories when we are sitting and also when we are moving. A decrease in muscle mass is linked with a progressive increase in fat mass, which results in changes in body composition. This is associated with an increased risk of insulin resistance in older people.

And what about oestrogen? Studies are mixed – some indicate it has an impact on weight gain and others say it has no role to play. More research is needed in this area. But we do know it has an impact on how fat is distributed around the body, promoting the move to surrounding the organs mentioned above.

Many women I talk to can't understand why they are heavier when they are doing the same exercise and eating the same diet as always – but what worked in the past won't work when you hit your forties. You need to tweak your habits and your approach. This means that weight loss takes much more effort than before.

We also often forget how important it is to keep blood sugar levels balanced. Think about a young child – we would never let them miss lunch, as we would pay dearly for it! We need to think the same way about ourselves and keep a closer watch on our blood sugar levels so we don't reach for the quick pick-me-up snacks like chocolate, which creates a catch-22 with weight gain. On top of all this, there are the sleep issues that many women face. When you don't get a good night's sleep, this can increase your craving for sugary foods, which perpetuates the cycle.

The important thing here is to understand that the rules change as we get older – not only in how to avoid gaining weight, but also in how to lose weight. So it's really important to try to keep on top of your weight in your forties and fifties. Excess weight, especially visceral fat, will put you at greater risk of type 2 diabetes, heart disease and many other illnesses.

I love running but the gym and me were never good buds. I've signed up with a personal fitness trainer, only one weight training session a week required for muscle tone and bone strengthening. We lose 40 per cent of muscle and bone density during the menopause so it's so important to keep on top of this. That's my story to date, not too unpleasant yet, but I do get anxious thinking about what may lie ahead.

– Christina

KEY FACTORS THAT LEAD TO WEIGHT GAIN

We can't put it all down to changing hormone levels, ageing and menopause. Other factors lead to weight gain, such as diet, stress, depression, low levels of activity, shift work, sleep issues, history of obesity, genetics, certain medications (it's a good idea to check any medication you are on) and chemotherapy. The place to start is to understand the role another key hormone, insulin, plays in this aspect of your health.

UNDERSTANDING INSULIN

Insulin, one of the most important hormones when it comes to both weight loss and gain, is responsible for fat storage. It is like a traffic controller and gatekeeper all in one. When you eat food, your body has to break it down to digest it and turn it into energy (fuel) for the body to run optimally. The body needs glucose for energy – but when it gets out of control, issues arise.

Glucose is a key source of energy and when you hear of blood sugar levels, that is the glucose in your blood. Carbohydrates provide glucose, which the body needs for energy, but when it gets out of control, issues arise. Being insulin sensitive is normal functioning. A person may move from this to insulin resistance, to pre-diabetes and finally type 2 diabetes.

Too much glucose in your body increases your blood sugar level. The body then kicks into action to remove the excess sugar and bring levels down again. To do this, it tells your pancreas to secrete insulin. Insulin acts like a key, having the ability to unlock the cells and let sugar in, allowing each cell in the body to create energy, to absorb the sugar from your blood. When there is excess sugar, insulin will send it to the liver, muscles and body fat, where it is then stored until needed – like having a back-up fuel tank for your car. While we always think of insulin with regard to blood sugar levels, it is also key in how our bodies absorb fats and proteins.

Due to wear and tear, the pancreas may produce more insulin than required. Over time, the insulin receptors in your body become less effective and 'insulin resistant' (the key can't open the locks to the cells, as they are worn). High levels of insulin in the body will cause inflammation, push the excess sugar to fat storage, impact your hormones and leave you at risk of type 2 diabetes. High levels of cortisol can trigger insulin production, which in turn may trigger the 'pregnenolone steal' and tip the balance to oestrogen dominance.

Your brain is hardest hit by the fluctuations in blood sugar levels, resulting in tiredness, low mood, and concentration and memory issues.

Diabetes, heart disease, stroke, dementia, cancer and premature ageing are all impacted by high insulin. Add testing for this with your doctor when needed – a fasting blood glucose or HbA1c test will show up impaired fasting glucose. Impaired fasting glucose, impaired glucose tolerance and diabetes all indicate insulin resistance, which can be present ten to fifteen years before any diagnosis. Up until then, the pancreas will have been working very hard to counteract the insulin resistance, but over time the pancreas will burn out. With type 2 diabetes, only 50 per cent of the pancreas remains functioning. Half the population are insulin resistant and 10 per cent develop diabeties. Increased urination, thirst and thrush are all common signs of diabetes. Sleep, movement, stress management and good food will help support healthy insulin production. In relation to your food habits, as outlined in Chapter 19, the key culprits are refined carbs, sugar, alcohol and highly processed foods with hidden sugars and other ingredients. Everything in moderation!

The most commonly asked question is: I'm exercising regularly but I'm not losing weight – why?

Weight management requires continuous effort as we get older. There is no magic bullet. It is a combination of the right food, movement, managing stress and lifestyle aspects, all of which will come together to help manage weight. As we've seen, insulin moves excess sugar to other parts of the body, primarily the muscles, liver and body fat. Your body has to work through each of these in turn when you exercise, making you use the sugar in your blood so the body won't be triggered to produce insulin to open those cells to store any excess. Where you have sufficiently low insulin levels, the body will eventually take sugar from fat storage, triggering weight loss. So movement has a direct impact on insulin resistance, which can support weight management. This is why a variety of movement is key, from cardio to resistance exercise. Integrating a mix of exercise, managing stress and eating the right foods is the starting point.

BMI AND WAIST MEASUREMENT

Body Mass Index (BMI) is the universal measure used by most medical professionals to assess body fat. It uses height and weight to determine where you fit on the ranking. BMI is not always reliable and does not take your body shape and build into account. Doctors may also look at waist measurements, which can be helpful to assess visceral fat (the fat deep inside that wraps your organs) – the location of body fat is key.

WHY IT IS IMPORTANT TO MANAGE YOUR WEIGHT

Gaining a lot of weight may make you more prone to illnesses like type 2 diabetes, cardiovascular disease and many other illnesses. Excess visceral fat (adipose tissue) is one of the key reasons women have an increased risk of heart disease. In many situations, it will also heighten your symptoms of menopause.

I have tried every diet under the sun, nothing worked. Every month I just gained more and more weight. I started to really dislike my body, and I was cross, angry and irritable the whole time. My best friend saw the toll this was taking on me and she was so encouraging. She got me to join a fitness class with her. Initially, I thought I would have a heart attack at each class, but then over the weeks things started to shift. I was losing weight! I also started to watch what I ate every day, and I know both steps have helped me so much to manage my weight. Having my friend support me was the turning point.

– Clare

STEPS YOU CAN TAKE

Adopt a daily movement habit

This can be whatever you like – whatever works for you. Try to build to at least thirty minutes of movement a day. As you get a routine going, look at weight-bearing exercises, as these are great for your body. Variety is the spice of life, especially when it comes to exercise. Remember, exercise should release those feel-good hormones and make you feel invigorated. See Chapter 18 for an in-depth look at daily movement.

Prioritise sleep

Why does sleep have such an impact on weight? The hormones insulin, cortisol and ghrelin come into play here. Lack of sleep results in increased cortisol levels, and cortisol promotes insulin resistance – back to that vicious cycle. The hunger hormone, ghrelin, will be higher after a night of no sleep. This means we will feel hungrier and will eat more, and chances are, too, we may reach for high-sugar foods, which give a quick fix but have a lasting impact on the body's flow of insulin. Both ghrelin and cortisol prompt the body to make more insulin, and that encourages the body to store the excess sugar as body fat.

On the plus side, a good night's sleep means you are burning excess fat while you sleep, as your body will tune into these reserves when needed to keep the body functioning. The longer you can be food-free at night time to the next morning the better. Ideally, you will have a few hours to digest any evening meal before bed, making sure your body goes into its reserves. Eating last thing at night means insulin will be high and hours will be spent digesting that late-night meal. Aim to stop eating two hours before bedtime – more if you can. A cup of herbal tea or glass of water can help bridge any hunger gap you may be feeling. Chapter 4 has many practical tips to help you establish good sleep habits.

Be mindful of *what* you are eating

Some people like to use pen and paper or an app to track what they eat on a daily basis – it helps them see where they are going astray. This can also help with eating mindfully, as often we eat out of boredom or habit. However, if tracking is a stressor for you, don't worry – just try to eat more fruit, vegetables and wholegrains and fewer processed foods in general. Often it can be better value and better for you to make your meals from scratch at home. (See Chapter 19 for more.)

Think about *when* you are eating

We know that we are what we eat. Next to this in importance is *when* we eat. Snacking and eating throughout the day will not benefit insulin levels and will put your body under constant pressure. When the body has no food to break down and process, it gets a break from insulin production. The body still has to work to do, though – it has to create energy to do whatever tasks and functions you are performing. With low levels of insulin circulating and more needed, the body can now look to its reserves.

Having structure around when you eat also benefits other aspects of your health, helping to reduce inflammation, promoting neuroplasticity and encouraging internal repair of any damaged cells (a process called autophagy). Deciding when your breakfast starts and when your eating finishes for the day are the key changes required, and then reducing snacking in between. For example, you might have breakfast at 8 a.m, lunch and dinner during the day, and a strict time for your final food intake. I find with many women that evening snacking is where they are caught out. They may manage well up until 3 or 4 p.m. and then things start to slip. If you have a clear goal in mind, it will make it easier and you will know what works best for you. If you're a shift worker, your times will vary compared to others.

The next part is eating when that hunger hormone (ghrelin) kicks in – listen to your body: that rumbling in your tummy is a good sign. This is all tied in with eating mindfully. During the day, eat when hungry as opposed to when you think you should or when you feel bored or other emotions strike.

Look after your gut

Gut health is an essential aspect of weight management and optimum health, with fibre being your best friend here (see Chapter 19 for more).

Read your labels

With everything you buy, study the labels. If there is an ingredient you're not familiar with, research it. Know what is going into your body. Just because a label says 'natural', it does not mean every aspect of it is. It could also mean it's derived from a natural source but many ingredients may have been added or stripped out along the way. Eating good food should not add additional financial pressure – rummage and be selective when picking your fresh produce.

Reduce alcohol consumption

Alcohol really is not a friend at this stage, as it puts more strain on your liver, which is already working hard. It can lower your body's ability to absorb much-needed calcium. It will also impact your sleep and generally results in your eating more too.

Avoid fad diets

There is no clinically proven menopause diet, and fad diets, for the most part, may just put more pressure on you. Eating well and exercising are the key habits to encourage. You want long-term sustainable change, not a quick fix that will rebound in another few months. Also, most fad diets wreak havoc on your blood sugar levels, which is a recipe for disaster in menopause!

Cut out sugar where you can

As we saw earlier, sugar intake and its impact on insulin is crucial in understanding how to manage weight. Our bodies need very little sugar and excess will trigger insulin resistance and encourage fat storage. And remember, many forms of sugar aren't obvious so, again, read your labels carefully.

* * *

Many people will follow all of the above steps but still struggle to manage their weight, in which case a multidisciplinary approach may be needed, ideally involving the GP and a dietitian. It is important to get the right support as you look to manage your weight in these years.

A lot of women tell me they hate their bodies and how heavy they have gotten. This saddens me. Weight and body changes are pretty much unavoidable later in life, but once we understand what is going on at perimenopause and what is happening at a physical level, we can understand why what worked before may not work now. You have to fit all the pieces of the puzzle together – understanding the role insulin plays, removing as much processed food as possible from your diet, looking at stress and sleep and keeping moving. Don't jump all in: start with small changes that will be lasting.

And the first step is accepting your body for where it is right now. Don't be cross with yourself; don't be unkind and harsh. Go gently. Respect the changes that are happening and build on the knowledge you have to change your daily habits to support you through these years. Small changes will reap long-term benefits.

11

Minding your heart

One woman dies every two hours, on average, in Ireland due to cardiovascular disease, and one woman every minute in the world. Cardiovascular disease is the leading cause of death for women worldwide. We are seven times more likely to die from heart issues than from breast cancer. Whenever I chat with friends about health, cancer always comes up, and as I started to research heart disease, I was stunned by the lack of awareness of how common a killer this is for women. Information is imperative here: taking preventative steps to manage your heart health starts with understanding what cardiovascular disease is and how it may impact you.

WHAT IS CARDIOVASCULAR DISEASE (CVD)?

Cardiovascular disease affects the heart, circulation and brain. It encompasses heart disease, peripheral vascular disease and stroke. The starting point is atherosclerosis: this is where plaques (fat, cholesterol and other ingredients) build up in the arteries, which makes them narrower. They are less elastic, less flexible and start to constrict. This impacts blood flow throughout your body and can result in blood pooling in an area and causing a clot. If this happens in the brain, it will cause a stroke. Angina, heart failure, arrhythmia (abnormal heart rhythm) and hypertension are other common forms of CVD.

How does it impact women?

As women reach fifty, the risk of heart disease starts to rise, with natural ageing and menopause at play here. We start to lose the protection our hormones gave us.

Women experience heart attacks differently to men – the classic movie scene of a man grasping his chest does not apply to a woman. Typically, a woman will experience pressure in the chest, back, neck, jaw or arm. It can feel a bit like a pulled muscle. This is accompanied by nausea, dizziness, tiredness, cold sweats and shortness of breath. These symptoms – which may be subtle initially – can mirror other conditions; the key difference is the ongoing nature of the symptoms. If they persist and last for twenty to thirty minutes, you need to be checked. Many of these symptoms overlap with those of menopause, but the important part is to seek help – it's better to be told all is fine than the alternative: a serious illness.

SIGNS OF HEART ATTACK IN WOMEN

Uncomfortable pressure in the centre of the chest, often lasting for a few minutes or coming and going
Back, neck, jaw, shoulder or stomach discomfort
Pain in one or both arms
Shortness of breath
Cold sweat
Nausea or vomiting
Dizziness or light-headedness
Unusual tiredness

What puts you at risk of CVD?

Women aged fifty to sixty are more prone. Smoking, sedentary lifestyle, weight gain, diet, alcohol use, type 2 diabetes and high blood pressure are common risk factors.

It is preventable?

The great news is yes! Cardio-vascular disease is 80 per cent preventable. There are practical steps you can take to ensure optimum heart health – see below.

WHAT IS A HEART PALPITATION?

This is when you feel a fluttering or pounding heartbeat: you will feel your heart racing and beating much faster than normal. Your heart can also skip a beat at intervals during palpitations. This intense feeling can extend from your chest up to your neck and throat. It can be extremely frightening to experience, even if just for a few minutes. In most cases, palpitations are not a sign of an issue with your heart but with other lifestyle factors. To make things trickier, they can often happen at the same time as a hot flush.

What can cause palpitations?

From my experience with the women I have worked with, lifestyle factors are the biggest cause – primarily chronic stress and anxiety. This is why I think we see palpitations so much in menopause: it is a time when anxiety is heightened, and the physical manifestation can be palpitations. The fall in oestrogen in these years also compounds the issue.

Other things that can cause palpitations are:

- Smoking
- Alcohol
- Caffeine
- Low blood sugar levels
- Low blood pressure
- Dehydration
- Overactive thyroid
- Irregular heart rhythms
- Some cough and cold medicines that contain pseudoephedrine

If the palpitations don't happen very often and only last a few seconds when they do occur, it will help to make some of the lifestyle changes outlined below. Especially, look at anxiety and stress – bear in mind, too, that palpitations can happen when you seem at your calmest but underneath, like the iceberg analogy, there is a lot going on. No matter what, be sure to check with your GP if you're in any way concerned.

STEPS TO PROTECT YOUR HEART HEALTH

Awareness

Be conscious of heart health: make sure to have your blood pressure and cholesterol checked annually, as this will flag any risk. Remember, high blood pressure shows no symptoms, hence it's called the 'silent killer'. It's very common for blood pressure and cholesterol to increase in the perimenopause years.

Stress

Ongoing chronic stress impacts all aspects of your health, and most importantly your heart health. Be honest with yourself here and look at the stresses in your life, bearing in mind that what is a stress for one person might not be for another. (See Chapter 12 for more on how to manage stress.)

Smoking

If you smoke, please talk to your doctor about ways to stop – it is no friend to you. Research suggests that women who smoke will have menopause earlier.

Sugar

Blood vessels have a lining called the endothelium, a layer of cells that are like smooth pebbles in a river. The blood flows over them easily, as they are smooth and flat. These cells are lined with fine hairs. The hairs, called glycocalyx, protect the cells from harm and damage. Too much sugar in the blood can damage this important layer of protection, and this can increase the risk of blood clots.

Alcohol and caffeine

Reduce and eliminate these if you can – either in excess will make the journey harder, and they are not heart healthy.

Exercise

Incorporate activity into your daily life – this will help you in many ways. Stress, anxiety and general health all benefit from daily exercise. It will lower blood pressure and help prevent insulin resistance. It doesn't have to be a marathon gym session, but a brisk walk or something you enjoy, and thirty minutes per day will help. One hour of movement per week can reduce the risk of heart attack and stroke by up to 70 per cent. Incorporate relaxation techniques like breathing, yoga and meditation into your life too. And don't forget that your heart is a muscular organ, so muscle-strengthening activities have a role to play here.

Sleep

Incorporate good sleep habits to try and ensure nourishing sleep. And remember that even resting will be a benefit to you – it's important that sleep itself does not become a stressor.

Menu

Optimise your intake of omega-3, magnesium and fibre-rich foods. Garlic is also excellent to support heart health. Eat more fruits, green vegetables and whole grains. Try to reduce salt and sugar. (For more, see Chapter 19.)

Blood pressure medication

Your doctor may prescribe blood pressure medication – this comes in many guises and beta-blockers are the most common.

HRT

The benefit of HRT is in starting it within the first ten years of menopause, as it promotes healthy arteries. The role of oestrogen within the heart is to help your blood vessels maintain their flexibility and not become inflamed – it simply keeps them healthy.

The NICE (National Institute for Health and Care Excellence) guidelines (evidence-based recommendations for health and care in England) state that:

- HRT does not increase cardiovascular disease risk when started in women aged under sixty.
- HRT with oestrogen alone is associated with no, or reduced, risk of coronary heart disease.
- HRT with oestrogen and progestogen is associated with little or no increase in the risk of coronary heart disease – estimated as being an additional five women per thousand.
- The risk of blood clots associated with HRT is greater for oral than transdermal preparations, so transdermal rather than oral HRT should be considered for menopausal women at increased risk of blood clots.

Statins

These are used to reduce high serum cholesterol. It's important to make an informed decision about their use for yourself, and their side effects must be taken into account: tiredness and muscle pain in the legs are common, while kidney failure and muscle breakdown are rarer symptoms. Unfortunately, women experience more side effects of statins than men.

CoQ10

As we get older, and especially from twenty years onwards, production of CoQ10 declines in the body. Levels have been found to be lower in those with existing heart conditions and with people using statins. CoQ10 can be found in meat, fish and nuts or a supplement.

Other

Plant sterols and niacin (B3) also play a valuable role in maintaining a healthy heart.

WHEN TO SEE YOUR DOCTOR

Keeping track of your heart health is very important throughout menopause, and this can be monitored through the following steps with your doctor:

- Looking at your family history.
- Checking your blood pressure – high blood pressure (hypertension) indicates a risk: it means your heart is having to work harder to pump blood around the body. Your doctor will monitor you over periods of time. Lifestyle and/or medication will reduce your risk.
- Doing blood work – HDL and LDL cholesterol are the key markers here. You want HDL to be high and LDL to be low. (High cholesterol can also indicate thyroid disease so it is important to rule that out.) Your triglycerides may also be checked – these are a type of blood fat essential for health.
- Checking for insulin resistance and type 2 diabetes, which are strong risk factors also.
- Possibly also requesting an ECG (to check your heart's rhythm and electrical signals) or a coronary calcium scan if you have risk factors for heart disease.

* * *

Future-proofing your heart health is crucial. The steps you take today will set you up for a happy heart in the years ahead – remember, 80 per cent of heart disease is preventable with lifestyle changes.

12

The psychological side of menopause

Nobody warns you about the psychological changes that come with menopause – a loss of confidence, creeping anxiety, a sense of approaching doom and doubting yourself about things you've never questioned before. And when it comes to mood swings, most of us have a story or two to tell. The good news is that it passes. Personally, I felt much stronger at the age of fifty-two, edging closer to menopause, than I felt at forty-five, in early perimenopause.

I firmly believe the psychological aspects of menopause are underrated and misunderstood, and they cause the most challenges for many women.

Perimenopause alters the way your brain functions. Because hormone receptors are situated in the brain, it stands to reason that when hormone levels vary and then start to decline, it may affect your mental health. These changing hormones, just as in puberty and in pregnancy, if you have experienced it, may make you feel more sensitive, more irritable and less tolerant than usual. I describe it as being more 'PMT like' in how you are feeling. Many women don't connect these changes with the start of the perimenopause years, and they worry about what is going on.

My body was in a constant heightened state of anxiety caused by rapidly plummeting hormones, yet I blamed myself for not being able to shake it off.

The psychological effects have been devastating also. Vicious mood swings where I veered from homicidal to suicidal. The urge to self-harm was incredibly strong – anything to feel something other than the rottenness I had become accustomed to.

Nobody understood and that is a very lonely place to be. My poor mother went through the same thing but had no words for it and no support from others.

– Fiona

THE MIDLIFE YEARS

In the 1960s, psychologist Elliott Jacques invented the term 'midlife crisis', which he applied to both men and women. Women's midlife has traditionally been viewed as a period of adjustment to loss, such as loss of identity, loss of loved ones, empty nest, fertility loss and loss of youth.

On the bright side, Jungian analyst James Hollis feels that midlife can be a time to reflect on one's life. It's also a good moment to pause, re-evaluate and reassess. He refers to midlife as the 'middle passage' rather than a crisis. Who are we apart from our history and roles played up to this point, Hollis asks. If there is a disconnect between women's inner sense of themselves and the personalities they feel they need to display, they might want to change in order to rediscover their true selves, reclaim their lives and find significance. To me, this is the opportunity of menopause, the opportunity for reconnection with ourselves. The Chinese see the word 'crisis' as having two components: danger and opportunity. And as the saying goes, 'In the midst of every crisis lies great opportunity.'

Germaine Greer argues that all women are forced to think about themselves in terms of how others and society see them until they reach midlife. For women in their forties, a shift occurs when they are startled into consciousness, such as by illness, the death of a loved one, divorce or the loss of a career. This is when women begin to question the purpose of life, as well as their own personal meaning, and when they desire to take control of their identities. Menopause also brings this reawakening.

Many women in their forties and fifties begin to feel less bound by cultural constraints, to see the importance of their own decisions and to become less defined by what is expected of them. Midlife is seen as a moment to tap into this potential and bring all aspects of our personalities together into a more complete, whole self.

This desire for change – bringing both positive and negative feelings – may partly explain the emotional rollercoaster, the sensation of being stuck, overwhelmed and the loss of sense of self. A catalyst, such as a psychological shift, is required for change to occur. The signs of midlife distress, according to James Hollis, should be welcomed, since they may eventually lead to a great desire for rejuvenation.

Menopause is change and reassessment

It's all about change – physical, spiritual, emotional. Every part of a woman's life is up for reassessing. Change brings regeneration and vigour, and with it comes the ability to choose. When women realise this, they become much more selective with their time and energy, using both wisely and letting go of what no longer serves them well.

This is the perfect period in life for women to gain self-confidence and become the best version of themselves. Menopause is a time to embrace your true self, to live in accordance with your values and the people that matter to you. Many women may be embracing their genuine selves for the first time, free of the responsibilities of the roles they have assumed up to this point. For women, menopause may be a very empowering and gratifying time in their lives.

Mindset

Be aware of your mindset toward your menopause and ageing. Ask yourself how you view the world and your place in it – do you have a positive outlook on life, an open or closed mindset? Our mindset and attitude play a significant role in all our life's outcomes. I believe if we can empower ourselves with knowledge and understand the challenges we may encounter, we can change the way we approach and experience this life stage. If we know what is ahead, we can decide how we look at the experience. Instead of worrying, we can move to embracing these years as an opportunity.

WHY THE EMOTIONAL UPHEAVAL IN MENOPAUSE?

The fall in hormones that happens in these years, primarily oestrogen and progesterone, may impact our psychological health. Oestrogen is a feel-good hormone – when our body has ample stores of it, all is well in our world. So when it starts to decline, we can experience low mood, anxiety and other general feelings of stress. Our resilience takes a hit and our 'bounce-back-ability' is off-kilter – we are knocked off balance. Progesterone and testosterone are also declining, which adds fuel to the fire.

Many of us suddenly feel unable to cope with situations that were never a problem before. We feel overwhelmed by simple aspects of day-to-day living. This can be frightening and undermine our confidence, and we may even assume that we are slowly losing control of our minds.

Some psychological symptoms may be related to physical changes brought on by the rebalancing of your hormones. Falling oestrogen levels can make you feel emotional; dehydration caused by sweats and hot flushes can cause panicky feelings; and the very common memory lapses can make you feel anxious that you are losing your memory and losing control, which impacts your confidence and self-esteem and adds to your daily stress.

The 'sandwich' years add to this, where you are possibly juggling kids, ageing parents, work, daily life and then your menopause on top.

Many women have spoken to me about this, and when they realise that their new-found sense of depression, anxiety and disquiet can be explained by menopause, they are immediately calmer and, as a result, more enabled to take charge of their lives and health again.

> The main symptoms I suffered with were crippling anxiety and insomnia, which had a profound impact on all areas of my life. I thought it was some sort of breakdown or depression, as we had moved back to Ireland after living abroad.
>
> Knowledge is key at this stage in our lives – I had given myself six months to live in my head! If I had been better informed that this was all normal, I wasn't dying or going crazy, I might have had an easier passage!
>
> – Sinead

DEPRESSION

Depression is a medical illness associated with persistent sadness, loss of hope, low energy and little interest in life. It is more than merely feeling sad: there can be feelings of utter despair, bleakness and a loss of joy. It is unfortunately very common, and women who have had depression in the past are more likely to experience a recurrence during these years. Menopause brings with it an increased risk of depression – anywhere from 19 to 41 per cent of women are impacted.

Serotonin is an important hormone in relation to your well-being and happiness levels. When oestrogen levels drop during menopause, serotonin levels drop as well. You may also be creating far more of the stress hormone, cortisol. High amounts of cortisol can compromise serotonin generation.

Experiencing many of the other symptoms of menopause can create the perfect storm for mood changes. It becomes a vicious cycle where loss of sleep due to stress or night sweats will lead to tiredness, triggering brain fog and concentration issues. And sleeping for less than six or seven hours each night is linked to depression worsening. As you saw in Chapter 4, ongoing sleep issues have an impact on your long-term health. Sleep is really the bedrock of thriving through menopause.

Poor food choices can then come on top of this, as you may reach for the easiest, quickest food. Then your moods are impacted – not just by loss of sleep but also by the food you're eating: irritability sets in, and your confidence and self-esteem take a hit, which invariably leads to low mood. Excess alcohol intake will also impact you greatly here.

This may all be exacerbated by your own past. Unresolved adverse childhood and life experiences may impact your susceptibility to feeling low. This may be further compounded if you don't have the right support through these years – from your family, work, friends, community and social interaction. Therapeutic support is crucial in this case.

Premenstrual depression, postnatal depression and menopausal depression are clinical manifestations of reproductive depression in women, linked to hormonal changes throughout the menstrual cycle, pregnancy and menopause. Knowledge is power, so be aware that if you were prone to earlier forms of hormonal-related depression, there is a higher chance you may experience it in your perimenopause years. Menopause transition, while offering a window of opportunity, is also a window of vulnerability, with that risk of depression being higher.

The key is to work with your doctor to understand whether your depression is part of your menopause or whether it is clinical depression. The good news is there is a lot you can do to support yourself, which we will look at in this chapter too.

I have bipolar disorder and have been on medication constantly for over twenty years. I have it well managed at this stage (thankfully) but have a few 'blips' here and there. About eight months ago, I noticed that my mood would go very low coming up to my period. It might last four or five days. Like magic, a few days after it would be as if nothing happened and I wouldn't even be able to tell you what I had been crying about the few days previous!

My GP trusts that I am very aware of my mood and suggested I try HRT. I was very afraid, as I couldn't predict how it may affect my mood. I'm on an oestrogen patch and progesterone tablet. Early days, but I feel it has made a difference.

– Olivia

ANXIETY

Anxiety is something most people will experience at some point in their life. Remember how you felt the night before the Leaving Cert? Anxiety is another word for worries, fears, feeling scared or frightened. It is a double-edged sword: we need anxiety and fear – these emotions are essential to basic human survival. Way back when we lived in caves, these emotions kept us alert to danger and were a form of protection, helping us to avoid predators or hazards in our environment. Now, these emotions keep us attuned to any potential threats – from a speeding car to a developing fever in our child.

But when these healthy fears get out of control, we need to take action. Developing a greater understanding of anxiety is the essential first step to reducing and dealing with these feelings. Research shows that women are twice as likely to be affected by and diagnosed with anxiety disorders as men are.

Menopause-onset anxiety is very common and can be one of the most difficult symptoms to cope with during this time of transition. Just knowing that it is common and that you are not alone can be immensely comforting, and being able to talk openly about your anxiety can be therapeutic. Anxiety is like a build-up of pressure in our minds. It is stating the obvious, but to alleviate this pressure we need to vent the anxiety.

Of all the symptoms of menopause, anxiety is the one I have encountered the most and that women are beginning to speak about more openly. Often, it's the first symptom women experience, starting in their early forties for natural menopause. So it's not the more common physical symptoms of the hot flush or the night sweats but the slow onset of anxiety creeping in that often marks the beginning of menopause.

Being highly anxious most of the time is emotionally and physically exhausting and leads to a whole host of additional symptoms. The symptoms of anxiety will range from immediate physical symptoms (such as raised blood pressure, rapid breathing, frequent urination) to long-term symptoms like headaches, insomnia, digestive issues and nausea. All of this can result in changes to our behaviour – avoidance, irritability, isolation, tiredness and anger.

The most common forms of anxiety in menopause are generalised anxiety, panic attacks, social anxiety and health anxiety.

> I was exactly forty-seven and four months when menopause hit me straight out of left field. From being a happy, successful, gregarious go-getter, I turned into a frightened kitten. I was terrified I would lose my livelihood, my marriage and my health. Having lost my dad before the pandemic, not able to visit the grave or village I was from 140 miles away, it was put down to stress and I was prescribed SSRIs. My friends and husband of ten months, who knew me so well, couldn't believe this, and as we couldn't identify the source of the crippling anxiety and sleepless nights, we all knew something else was going on.
>
> – Ciara

STRESS

We feel stress when we feel threatened or under pressure. When you are in a situation you have no control over, you may feel stress – many of us felt that during Covid. The problem is that often we are in this state when there is no actual threat, but the body perceives one and so triggers our fight-or-flight response.

Through menopause we also become more sensitive to physical aspects of life – noise, lights, food – and this leads to emotional sensitivity, also triggering an increased sensitivity to stress. Things happen, life happens: what is important is to become aware of how you and your body respond.

What's happening in your body

As we learned in Chapter 8, oestrogen, which is produced in the ovaries and locally in the brain, has a big impact on our brain. It aids in the increase of blood flow, the optimal functioning of the brain and the improvement of brain connectivity. When it comes to our moods, oestrogen increases serotonin activity.

Your beautiful brain comprises three regions: the brainstem, the limbic system and the cerebral cortex. The brainstem is responsible for your body's automatic functions like heart rate and temperature regulation. The limbic system is responsible for emotion, learning and memory, a key component being the amygdala, which processes fear and emotional memory.

The amygdala triggers the all-important stress response. The HPA (hypo-thalamic–pituitary–adrenal) axis is then activated: this is where your hormones and neurological system communicate. A feedback system exists between these three glands, with the hypothalamus and pituitary being the overseers of the levels of cortisol in your blood. Too high or too low and the brain sends a message to the adrenals to produce more or less. When your adrenal glands release cortisol, it travels through the blood to all parts of your body. Almost every cell in your body contains cortisol receptors, so its effects are far reaching. At the same time, your body triggers the production of adrenaline, which will heighten the stress response. These are the hormones that kick you into action when stress hits: they tell your heart to pump faster and get you ready to run from danger. And when the stress response kicks in, anxiety heightens. As we've seen earlier, too much cortisol has several effects in the body, including impacting serotonin production, and this decline makes you more susceptible to feeling low.

The cerebral cortex is the last component of the brain, and it is responsible for making sense of your experiences and interactions with the outside world. The brain's response to everyday events may impact your psychological health and, for many, it comes under additional pressure in menopause.

The production of oestrogen diminishes as a woman advances from peri-menopause to menopause. Because oestrogen is a chemical signal, it influences not only progesterone (remember the hormonal dance they perform) but also other hormones in your body, including serotonin. When your serotonin levels

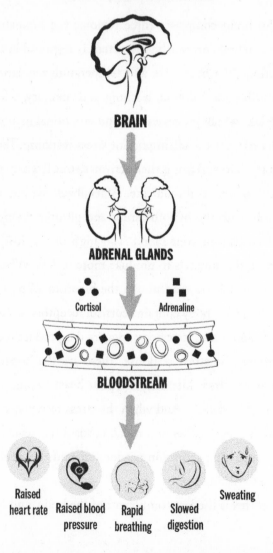

YOUR STRESS RESPONSE

BRAIN

ADRENAL GLANDS

Cortisol   Adrenaline

BLOODSTREAM

Raised heart rate   Raised blood pressure   Rapid breathing   Slowed digestion   Sweating

are low, it affects the hormones produced by your thyroid, adrenal glands and, most crucially, pituitary glands, which manufacture serotonin.

Cave people were only concerned with basic survival needs and staying alive. Today we live in much safer times (in terms of basic survival) but our brains have not evolved yet to distinguish between manageable everyday fears and big threats to our safety. They equate our modern daily challenges with the life-threatening challenges that our early ancestors experienced. Today, the challenges we face are more complex, and our brains can read a situation as life-threatening, which triggers a stress response, releasing adrenaline, and this sends off a fear signal, which releases the fight–flight–freeze hormones, which trigger the mental and physical changes. Our body is then in a heightened state of alertness and the mind becomes very sharp and focused. Cortisol is invading and taking over our body. Once the event is over, the body slowly returns to normal (albeit exhausted).

People frequently suffer episodes of hyper- or hypo-arousal during times of acute stress. Hypervigilance, anxiety and/or panic and racing thoughts are common symptoms of hyperarousal – the fight-or-flight reaction. Feelings of emotional numbness, emptiness or paralysis can be caused by hypo-arousal – the freeze reaction.

There is a psychological term called the 'window of tolerance': when a person is within their tolerance window, their brain is functioning properly and can process the world well. Without feeling overwhelmed or withdrawn, that person is likely to be able to reflect, think clearly and make calm decisions. When the window of tolerance collapses and your body closes down to the outside world, the traditional fight-or-flight reaction may alter to that of the freeze response.

Each person's tolerance window is different. The environment can also influence this: people are more likely to stay within their window when they feel safe and supported. A traumatic or otherwise unfavourable event may have the effect of pushing a person out of their tolerance window.

The adrenals and cortisol

Excess cortisol coursing through your body takes a toll. It will make you feel wired, unable to relax, jittery, nervous and more. The symptoms of excess cortisol will remind you of many perimenopause symptoms too – anxiety, depression, mood swings, tiredness, digestive issues, headaches, heart disease, high blood pressure, concentration issues, sleep disturbances, weight gain and low libido.

The adrenal glands produce cortisol and adrenaline, but they also produce oestrogen, testosterone (both via a precursor hormone) and progesterone. While earlier in life this is in smaller amounts than in the ovaries, at menopause they become the main producer of these hormones, so we want them to be healthy as we get older. However, often by perimenopause age, the adrenal glands may be depleted and not functioning as well as we want. In this state, the priority of the adrenals will be to produce whatever amount of cortisol the body needs, and the sex hormones take a back seat. The result is exacerbated symptoms of menopause and adrenal fatigue symptoms. (There are also conditions, for example Addison's disease, where the body does not make enough cortisol.)

Learning to manage your stress will help keep your adrenal glands healthy – one impacts the other. Happy, healthy adrenals will produce good hormones, and this will lead to a more positive menopause experience.

The other side of cortisol

I don't want to make cortisol out to be the bad guy. It has other roles, like managing metabolism, blood sugar, the circadian rhythm (vital for sleep), your immune response and inflammation. It is commonly referred to as a steroid hormone, which your body makes to help fight inflammation when needed. At the right levels, cortisol can contribute to good memory, motivation and decreased sensitivity to pain.

MENOPAUSE AND SUICIDE

Both the UK and Ireland experience female suicide rates at their highest with women of menopausal age. We cannot ignore this. If you are struggling, please reach out, and contact your GP, so you can get the right support and treatment (see Resources).

NEURODIVERSITY

ASD, ADHD and dyslexia are some common neurodevelopmental conditions and, to date, research is limited but does tell us that ADHD and similar conditions can result in heightened menopause symptoms, especially in relation to the psychological aspects of menopause.

TRANSGENDER HEALTH

To date, limited research has been conducted in the area of trans and non-binary health and the menopause, and the challenges trans and non-binary people can experience both physically and psychologically. Further research is needed to support people going through all forms of menopause from a diverse and inclusive perspective.

STRESS IN THE WORKPLACE

In today's world the workplace can take many guises – it can be in the home or outside. The symptoms of menopause can impact on your work, particularly anxiety. Sitting in a meeting, surrounded by peers, you hit those dreaded foggy moments and start to question yourself, then your mind takes over and one brief lapse of memory turns into something bigger. You may question your right even to be at the table. You may question your ability to do your job – the job you have been doing for years and are excellent at. Recognising what is happening and why will help you to cope with this.

WHAT YOU CAN DO

Understanding the body's response to psychological distress provides the key to unlocking how to deal with it. View your body's response as an ally, not as an enemy. For example, before I do a public event I always feel a mixture of anxiety and excitement. My trick is to focus my thoughts on the excitement, rather than the anxiety – the scales could tip either way if I don't keep my mind in check.

The human body has evolved to handle stress and anxiety in dangerous situations, but when stress and anxiety are persistent and constant, our bodies feel drained – emotionally and physically. When we feel low and vulnerable, we start to worry more about our health, and that provokes further anxiety, which in turn creates more exhaustion – and soon enough, a vicious cycle is keeping you in a state of anxiety lockdown.

Becoming aware of this process may help you understand why you feel like you do, and understanding can take the fear away. When you fear something, fretting about it blows it out of proportion, and so this fear begins to overtake your life and gains control.

Don't repress your anger

Anger comes in blasts like a blazing furnace: rage over someone in your usual parking spot, food on the wrong shelf in the fridge. The smallest things can trigger the mightiest of outbursts, without you understanding why you reacted in this way. Anger is a valid emotion, an energy like all our other emotions. When emotions are repressed because we don't want to validate them, this becomes problematic. Anger is OK, emotions are OK. Repression of emotions is not good for you. Your anger can be small or it can be volcanic, but the important step is to acknowledge it and work with it.

Pushing anger down and ignoring it, trying to step on it and conceal it, will not do you any favours. Repressed anger may lead to depression and illness. There are physical and mental consequences of suppressing emotions – it causes stress in your body. Being open to your feelings moves you closer to your real self. This is what your menopause wants: it wants to bring you home to you. For many women, there are years of repressed emotions, especially anger, waiting to be released – menopause blows the lid off the pressure cooker. Talking about your emotions is your expression of how you are feeling and will support you as you navigate these emotions. Often this can mean dealing with past issues that are as yet unresolved.

You may need support through this, and I would highly recommend counselling. There are many ways to access counselling, either through your workplace employee assistance programme (EAP), local services or privately.

Past adversity or trauma

Perimenopause raised the issue of my mum's passing almost thirty years ago that I never dealt with. I never grieved her. I don't know and probably never will if it was connected, but I'm pretty sure it was.

– Mags

Sadness at the loss of years, loss of fertility and the general loss that menopause brings can be interwoven with the resurgence of past traumas too. It is not easy. This can be a time of grief in many guises, but it can also be a time of empowerment. How we view it unlocks the experience.

Menopause attracts unresolved past issues like a bee to honey. The end result is sweet but the process can have a real sting in its tail. It is a deeply psychological time but one that, with the right attention, can bring growth and renewal. That's easy to say, but if you are a survivor of trauma (and, remember, what is traumatic for one person may not be for another – it does not have to be a major event), the reawakening of these emotions is downright petrifying. Your menopause shines a light on these unresolved issues and wants them decluttered before moving you on to the next chapter of freedom. Sometimes these trauma symptoms, even when they feel counterproductive, are longing for expression, to be felt, validated and ultimately released. And trauma comes in many guises, from relationships throughout your life that need to be processed to events that happened.

It's as if the first half of life needs to be addressed before we can enter the second half.

A few years ago I did a panel interview on sexual health. I expected to chat about libido and other physical aspects. What I was not prepared for was the stories women shared of past abuse and how they were reliving it vividly in menopause. Bessel van der Kolk talks of the 'unbearable heaviness of remembering' – to me, this sums it up perfectly.

It is crucial to have the right support when working through past trauma, so ensure you find a therapist experienced in this area, as it is highly complex and should never be about retraumatising you. Delving into this is beyond the scope of these pages, but nevertheless it's important to be aware that it may come up in these years, and working with a specialist in trauma is essential. (See Resources for more.)

> I think it would be hugely beneficial for women (and men) to realise that grief is no respecter of hormones and hormones are no respecter of grief.
>
> The symptoms of a grieving woman aged forty-five-plus can be very similar to that of perimenopause, and thus perimenopausal symptoms can be overlooked/dismissed. In a society where we still have to keep striving to increase knowledge and keep demanding more recognition for the life stage of perimenopause/menopause and all that entails, I see hope that a more authentic and realistic perspective of grief and ageing can happen in tandem with the power of personal stories about the menopause.
>
> – Jillian

Crucial care

Crucial care – minding you – is taking care of your mind and body and soul the way you might expect a physician or therapist to, except that you administer it yourself, equipped with the knowledge and diligence to practise it every day. It is about emotional health as much as physical health. It is non-negotiable if you want to deal effectively with your menopause. Being compassionate and kind to yourself is crucial. We will discuss this more in Chapter 22.

Slow life down – six daily habits

Do not underestimate the impact of your emotions on your energy levels. We have already talked about anxiety and adrenaline – how, when the body has been processing adrenaline, it can often leave it deflated and tired. Exhaustion, tiredness and yawning are all common with generalised anxiety and can often result in anxiety being mistaken for depression (although one can lead to the other). So while insomnia and hot flushes may leave you feeling tired, so too can the mental weariness that accompanies anxiety. Here are some things you can try daily to give yourself a break:

Be present: Stay present where you are right now – 'Right here, right now, I am fine.' Don't stray into the past, ruminating; don't worry about the future – where you are right now is safe.

Breathing: Practise simple breathing techniques to quickly quell anxiety. Take deep slow breaths to ground you and self-soothe during those periods of self-doubt and uncertainty.

Be outdoors: Stand outside for five minutes, regardless of the weather, and just breathe it all in. You probably already know about the physical health benefits of walking, and maybe about some of the psychological benefits of being in green open spaces. But there's another wonderful benefit of walking that's perhaps less commonly understood, and that's something called 'optic flow'. As you move forward, the world flows around you and your eyes naturally track left to right. This 'optic flow' and eye movement have a calming effect on the nervous system by reducing activity in the amygdala – the part of the brain most often associated with fear and anxiety. You've probably already experienced this if you've ever stomped out of the house for a walk and returned feeling a lot calmer!

Practise mindfulness as much as you can in your day. A great place to start is mindful eating (see Chapter 18) – 90 per cent of your serotonin production comes from your gut, so placing emphasis on good food is key. Protein foods containing tryptophan, such as milk and oats, are important, as this is part of the production process for serotonin.

Unplug from technology and all that fear of missing out. Read a book instead or listen to a funny podcast – it's all about doing something nice for yourself.

Find somebody to talk to: be social. Having support is essential, and that can be through your family or friends. But make sure and talk to your doctor about how you are feeling too.

Your warrior kit

Your journey through menopause is like crossing a river on stepping stones – there may be jumps and slips along the way. Here are some practical tools to support your emotional health in these years:

- Happy playlist: you can never go wrong listening to music. Make a playlist of music that you love or that calms you. You can also listen to a meditation app.
- Exercise: hit the road, the gym or the pool – exercise is both distraction and antidote (see Chapter 18).
- Nourishment: low blood sugar levels can trigger anxiety, so don't forget to eat (see Chapter 10).
- Chewing gum: chewing calms the jaw muscles and, while you may not have even noticed they were tense, this may bring some relief.
- Supplements: magnesium, vitamin D, vitamin C, the B vitamins, turmeric, L-theanine, GABA, saffron extract and 5-HTP can be helpful. Investigate herbs like maca, ashwagandha, lemon balm and rhodiola. (See

Chapter 16 for more information.)

- Hydration: always keep a bottle of water with you.
- Notebook: keep one with you so you can jot down some notes on how you feel and any symptoms that might be related – you can use your menopause journal, if you're keeping one.
- Wipes/tissues: these are helpful to have on hand if you are prone to perspiring.
- Affirmations: these are short positive statements you can repeat to yourself to help bring calmness and to reinforce the importance of positive self-talk. Keep some in your notebook or on your phone, and when a wobbly moment happens, hit repeat. Examples I like to use are:

  » I'm doing the best that I can.
  » I'm only human.
  » I am enough.
  » This too shall pass.
  » Feel the fear and do it anyway.
  » I am not this feeling.
  » This feeling cannot hurt me.

Counselling, psychotherapy and CBT

For many people, therapy, which provides a secure non-judgemental environment for people to have additional support, can be of great benefit. With the support of a mental health professional, you can often establish contact with your emotions without becoming overwhelmed and distressed. It is a safe, supportive environment, and a therapist will go at your pace to ensure no added stress.

Cognitive behavioural therapy (CBT) can help you manage your behaviours by changing the way you think and behave. CBT is most commonly used for anger management, anxiety and depression, but can be useful for other mental and physical health problems.

Medical options

Please talk to your doctor about how you are feeling and ensure you get the support you need. Also focus on your food, sleep, exercise and stress management.

HRT and other non-hormonal medications can be discussed with your doctor. HRT is often used to treat severe perimenopausal depression. Antidepressants should not be the first route for menopause, but they may provide invaluable support when the clinical picture shows the need for them.

The 6 Ms of menopause

These are designed to support all aspects of your health in menopause and future-proof your body. Each aspect will support your mental and emotional health also (see Part 4).

* * *

Life is a rollercoaster, full of ups and downs, twists and turns. We have all had challenges to deal with, and we are all bruised in some way from life. You may not realise it, but you are on a journey now – you are learning, changing, healing at some level or other. You are on a path of self-discovery. You are at the helm, charting your course through the rough seas, and with the right support you will reach the calmer waters of contentment and empowerment that menopause can bring.

13

Menopause at work

Women work throughout their lives, for many from a young age into later life, and that may be in the home or outside. Today, there are more women in the workplace than ever before, and the 45–64 age group is the fastest-growing labour force. Women daily are juggling home life, work and much more. The 'sandwich generation' has become a common term for this age group, with families and everyday life a constant juggle for many. Research into workplaces often focuses on the 'unencumbered' workforce – those with few to no responsibilities outside their jobs – and most workplaces are tailored to these workers, who are mainly male, leading to a gender data gap. Women are generally encumbered, working many unpaid hours outside the traditional workplace.

To top it all off, then comes menopause. In the midst of burning saucepans (let's be honest, we've all burnt at least one!), hot flushes and intense brain fog, work is still there. Menopause has no boundaries – it invades all aspects of our lives, and work is the place many women find the most challenging. It's not just yourself you have to think of: it's all those relationships intertwined – managers, co-workers, clients and many more.

Something has to give.

THE DISCRIMINATORY TABOO OF MENOPAUSE

Women aged forty to fifty tend to be at the prime of their careers when the menopause chapter starts. Years of wisdom and knowledge gained from working makes them instrumental in the workplace. However, many are now faced with the unknown experience that is menopause. Add to this the daily stress of juggling all the aspects of a woman's life, and the stress can become unmanageable.

Regardless of where you work, managing your menopause symptoms at work can present many challenges. The Faculty of Occupational Medicine in the UK states that eight out of ten menopausal women are in work. The trend is growing for women to stay longer in their careers, which means more women will transition through menopause in work, so it is imperative that this sensitive subject is addressed openly by workplaces and that women are supported throughout these years.

WELLNESS WARRIOR SURVEY

Understanding how menopause impacts a woman in her working day is key. In 2021, I conducted a survey of six hundred women about menopause in the workplace, which revealed the most challenging symptoms that impact women in their working day. And four out of five of those were psychological. These are the symptoms I strongly believe are most misunderstood and underrated for the far-reaching impact they have on a person's life. From the physical to the emotional effects, a key impact is loss of confidence and self-esteem.

According to the survey, almost one in three women had considered giving up their job due to menopause, with 70 per cent saying they would not discuss menopause with their managers. Alarmingly, 34 per cent of women had taken time off for menopause-related reasons, but 86 per cent were not comfortable telling their employer why. Sadly, more than two-thirds had never utilised their employee assistance programme (EAP), which is a shame, given the benefits and confidentiality this offers.

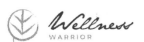

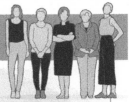

MENOPAUSE & YOUR WORK
2021 SURVEY RESULTS

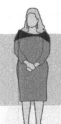

62% said menopause had a moderate impact on their work.

18% said it had an extreme impact on their work.

70% would not discuss with their manager, and for **49%** the key reason was lack of understanding

34% had taken time off due to menopause symptoms but **86%** were not comfortable telling their employer why

31% said that it was too sensitive a subject

96% would like menopause training & resources in their workplace

78% would like to see in-house manager training

49% would like an in-house support group with work colleagues

Three-quarters reported working from home during COVID had helped, with **more than half** being anxious about the return to the workplace.

ALMOST FOUR-FIFTHS of respondents feel it is still a taboo subject in the workplace.

MORE THAN TWO-THIRDS of respondents have never utilised their EAP programme.

PRACTICAL CHANGES WOMEN WOULD LIKE
69% a rest room or quiet space
49% the ability to work from home
48% access to a fan
31% wider food choices in the canteen
25% shower facilities
22% uniforms in non-synthetic material

© wellness warrior 2021

www.wellnesswarrior.ie

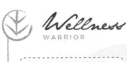

MENOPAUSE & YOUR WORK
2021 SURVEY RESULTS

TOP 5 SYMPTOMS WOMEN SAY IMPACT THEIR WORK:
- Brain Fog **77%**
- Anxiety **65%**
- Loss of confidence **60%**
- Insomnia **47%**
- Aches and pains **46%**

MAIN SUPPORTS BEING UTILISED
Supplements **64%**
Exercise **47%**
Mindfulness/Meditation **42%**
HRT **41%**
Other therapies **22%**
Talk therapies **17%**
Antidepressant **14%**

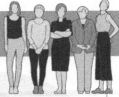

95% SAID THEIR WORKPLACE HAD NO MENOPAUSE GUIDANCE OR POLICY, while only about 1/3 of workplaces had a mental health policy.

ALMOST ONE IN THREE were considering giving up their job due to menopause.

With over **200 comments** made, the overriding emphasis was on education, awareness and support being needed in the workplace and across society.

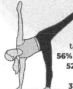

TOP 5 LIFESTYLE CHANGES MADE
71% started taking supplements
56% increased exercise
52% dietary changes
32% sleep habits
31% reduced caffeine

ADDITIONAL THINGS WOMEN WOULD LIKE TO SEE IN WORK:
Stand-up desks
Ability to ask for more breaks
Control of temperature
Cold water available
Caught-out kits

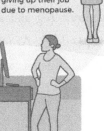

© wellness warrior 2021

www.wellnesswarrior.ie

Brain fog

This symptom tops the poll, with 77 per cent of women stating that brain fog was their biggest challenge at work. Brain fog is a heavy hitter for menopause in the workplace, encompassing memory loss, concentration issues and a feeling of a lack of clarity. It has a knock-on impact on confidence, self-esteem and anxiety. I have worked with countless women in various roles – factory workers, lawyers, nurses, retail assistants, teachers – who have all experienced the extremely unsettling issue that is brain fog. Many women in management roles found this to be the most challenging symptom, as it affects their ability to think clearly and retain facts and figures, impacting their capacity to problem-solve and work under pressure.

Anxiety

In general, anxiety impacts women more than men, which is why stress management is an essential part of menopause. The workplace can exacerbate this symptom. Great strides have been made in relation to mental health in general, but the area of emotional and mental health in menopause is vastly understated. The menopause years can be hectic for many women, and work becomes more challenging, which worsens and increases stress, giving rise to anxiety. This comes up in all workplaces. Support is key and a great starting point is your EAP.

Loss of confidence

Both brain fog and anxiety lead to loss of confidence, affecting 60 per cent of respondents. At menopause, your world starts to change due to hormonal upheaval. This has a direct impact on confidence, and many women struggle with this both at work and in their personal lives.

Sleep issues

In the survey, 47 per cent of respondents reported sleep issues. Loss of sleep due to hormonal changes or night sweats will impact your energy levels the next day. Ongoing tiredness will reflect in performance at work on a daily basis. Feeling tired will also impact levels of patience, mood and, most importantly, resilience. This will directly affect relationships with work colleagues. Insomnia will also cause brain fog, memory issues, increased stress levels and changing moods. A vicious circle!

Aches and pains

These affected 46 per cent of women and can be very challenging depending on the role being performed. A sedentary role adds an extra toll and, conversely, if a woman is standing all day, this again exacerbates the issue. Looking at women's experience of menopause by role is an essential starting point to providing support at work.

LEGAL ASPECTS OF MENOPAUSE

The Employment Equality Act of 1998–2015 incorporate employees' protection against discrimination. Nine protected grounds are set out in this legislation. The aim is to protect both human rights and equality in Ireland. Covered in this are equal opportunities, equal pay and the establishment of safe conditions of employment. Practical reasonable adjustments are also covered here. All employers have a responsibility to ensure the workplace is a safe place to work. This is why risk assessments have a part to play, especially if you have returned to work after surgery or treatment causing early menopause – your role ideally should be reviewed in light of any changes to your personal circumstances.

Menopause in its own right is not a disability. However, in some instances under case law it has been classed as such, given the ongoing nature and severity of symptoms and impact on a person's life.

A NEW OCCUPATIONAL HEALTH ASPECT

I've spoken in hundreds of workplaces, both in Ireland and globally, and the conversation is always the same. Employers are eager to understand what menopause is and how best they can support their employees. I have been thrilled to see many different companies and all kinds of organisations supporting this conversation. This needs to continue and, indeed, needs to be embedded within workplace guidelines, policies and procedures. Menopause needs to be accepted for the occupational health issue it is, just like pregnancy. And while not every woman, by choice or by circumstances, may experience pregnancy, all women will experience menopause.

Supporting menopause cannot be a 'flash in the pan' – one awareness session is not enough to cover menopause in a supportive manner. Full organisational workplace-wide support, with multiple channels available, is the way forward – from senior management to line managers to embedded policy changes.

Every single symptom of menopause you experience will have an impact on your daily life at work. The role you are performing at work may exacerbate your symptoms – for example, if you are a nurse, working with chronic sleep deprivation is going to be a hard burden to carry. If you work in retail and you are experiencing aches and pains, being on your feet all day can be distressing.

Employees deserve to feel supported and acknowledged by their employers during the transition that is menopause and how that transition impacts their working life. Ideally, we want to see workplaces raising the subject of menopause, as opposed to placing the onus on employees. We want to continue to shatter the silence around this topic and promote a culture of openness.

The number of menopause-related tribunal cases based on UK figures is on the increase, with more women feeling empowered to flag unfair working conditions and unfair dismissal (and these are just the ones that go to court – many more are settled outside of court).

I always did well at work. And then I just started to struggle. I couldn't keep on top of my work, I started to get anxious. I wasn't sleeping at night and was having night sweats. I was up several times a night changing. I dragged myself to work every day. I felt like a zombie. I put on weight, I wasn't eating well, my memory was gone to pot. And every day I was anxious. I lost all my confidence and just went into a shell.

– Anne

A SUPPORTIVE WORKPLACE

Menopause needs three things in the workplace: support, education and understanding.

Being a menopause-supportive workplace is being an inclusive workplace where all forms of menopause are supported. If you want to create and promote a diverse workplace that reflects the social community, the first step is to make your workplace a safe place for employees to openly raise and discuss personal issues – menopause is a key one.

In my experience of working with HR (human resources) managers and employers, the positive feedback they get from introducing and championing the topic and providing education sessions is second to none. Openly supporting menopause makes employees feel supported and acknowledged by their employers.

Sheryl Sandberg, ex-CEO of Facebook, stated that she found her work at Google challenging when pregnant, and her daily walk from the car park to the office took its toll. After several months, she approached one of Google's founders, informing him that they needed a pregnancy parking arrangement, ideally at the front of the building. It took her to experience pregnancy before she could see the need for this change within the workplace.

Policy change and supportive menopause policies in the workplace need to come from senior management down, and ideally more senior women need to come forward and raise awareness of these issues. I imagine many women in Google are thankful for Sheryl's policy change for pregnancy. It will be interesting to see what changes menopause can bring.

While it won't always be feasible, and most likely will depend on the field or type of business you work in, we also need to, as much as possible, empower ourselves, give ourselves permission to talk openly about menopause and not sweep the conversation under the carpet. Acknowledge the hot flush when it happens – don't hide it. Put your hand up to brain fog when it strikes – make the symptoms a normal part of life. This is the key to shattering the taboo and starting the menopause conversation in work and all aspects of life. I know this is not easy – it takes an openly supportive work environment for you to feel empowered to take this step and freely discuss menopause.

Practical support in the workplace can include menopause policies, guidance, surveys, reasonable adjustments, education and training, to name just a few.

> When I was about fifty, I felt I was going through a personality change. A big shift happened. I started to feel like I was losing control of myself. I grew extremely anxious and became aware of a low feeling. I thought I was getting depressed, I started to have negative thoughts, and a real sense of gloom came over me. This wasn't me. I have always been a bubbly, fun-loving person, outgoing, sociable and hard-working. Capable and confident too.
>
> I started to lose confidence in myself and was full of self-doubt. I felt like a poor mum, a poor wife, and I started to feel incapable of doing my job, telling myself that I was rubbish, my skills were outdated and I didn't fit in any more.
>
> – Anonymous

WHERE TO FIND SUPPORT AT WORK

Possible areas within your workplace to look for support are:

- Direct line manager
- Occupational health nurse

- HR representative
- EAP
- Menopause advocate or champion, if one exists in your organisation

How to open the conversation with your manager

Your direct manager may not have the same awareness or experience of menopause as you do, so it's important to have a simple, straightforward process to achieve a successful conversation with them when you're looking for support for menopause symptoms.

Awareness: Make your manager aware that you would like to speak to them about your menopause symptoms. This may be an email which states: 'I would like to meet with you next week to discuss some menopause symptoms I am experiencing and how I feel they are impacting my workday.' Or it may be a quick conversation where you say to your manager, 'I'd love to have a chat with you next week about my menopausal symptoms.' The important thing here is that you are giving your manager some time before you have the conversation. This allows them to do some research and gain some understanding to ensure they can have the conversation in a manner that will benefit you both. If you don't feel comfortable talking to your manager about this subject, see who else you can speak to – perhaps a colleague in HR or an occupational health nurse.

Prepare and have a solution: When the meeting is scheduled, do some prep work. Think about the main symptoms that impact your working day. For the initial meeting, one symptom is enough. For example, if you're experiencing hot flushes throughout the day and are working in an area under direct sunlight, you might request a change of position. When you present an issue or a challenge for you, have in mind what the solution could be. Your manager may not be overly familiar with the symptoms of menopause, so having a possible solution is essential.

Menopause guidance/policy: Check if your workplace has a policy in place. If there is none, see if there is a mental health policy, which may cover some aspects of the symptoms you are experiencing.

Notes: If you are experiencing some concentration issues, it is helpful to have some notes jotted down before the meeting so you can run through your key concerns.

Role play: Practise the conversation in front of the mirror or with your partner, a friend or work colleague. It will help reduce any nerves or anxiety you may feel about the meeting. Also, use it as an opportunity to look at various outcomes. This will help you prepare for possible scenarios that your manager may discuss with you. Another great option is to record your role play and watch it back. Doing this will make you feel more confident and in control of the conversation when it happens.

Breathe: A few minutes before the meeting, do a breathing exercise to prepare and calm yourself. Have your notes and water ready. Remember, you are here for support and your manager will (ideally) want to support you too.

Time: In the meeting, you might agree to changes that are easy to make quickly; however, there may be other solutions that take longer to implement, so do give your manager some time to come back to you.

Follow up: Agree on a date for you to catch up and monitor progress.

The aim of the meeting is for you to get support and practical solutions for the changing symptoms that may be impacting on your workday. This is an opportunity for you and your manager to work together to support you through your menopause journey. Approaching it in a united way is of huge benefit to both of you.

If you follow the above steps and do not get the desired outcome, it may be time to speak with a HR representative.

MAINTAINING RELATIONSHIPS AT WORK

You may feel butterflies in your stomach; you may feel a sense of dread and anticipation. And this is because you don't know how your colleagues will react to raising the subject of menopause – for many people, the symptoms and experiences may be too personal, and colleagues may not feel comfortable discussing how you are feeling. But having a trusted confidante at work will provide much-needed support, and while the initial conversation may feel awkward (you may even throw yourself into a hot flush at the thought of it), the end result can only be positive.

I'm not proposing that you go all intense with your work colleagues on the subject, merely open it up. It could be as simple as, when you experience a hot flush, saying, 'Oh, here's another hot flush.' Many women say that once they raise symptoms they're experiencing with a colleague, for the most part they find their colleagues have experience of something similar.

So grab a coffee, sit down with a trusted colleague and slowly open the conversation. This will allow you to build your support in the workplace. Chances are your colleague may be experiencing the same thing, or their partner may be, and you would both benefit from shared conversations.

Out of nowhere I began to experience anxiety, exhaustion and a complete lack of motivation, which led to me to feeling angry and very frustrated because I've been self-employed for almost twenty years and I'm known for my high energy.

When I finally surrendered from fighting my feelings, I found compassion for myself. I slept when I needed to, which was a lot; I allowed my tears to flow and this could happen without much warning; and I spent lots of time in nature hiking. The world didn't stop revolving because I stepped out for a while. I used the time to learn about myself, especially my emotions. I have equipped myself with techniques and tools to help me let go of what's not serving me and keep my peace. I do my best to stay in FLOW in business and work from inspired action instead of pushing through.

– Amanda Delaney, mindset mentor

RUNNING YOUR OWN BUSINESS

So what do you do when it's just you? If there's one thing I've learned from building my business from a blog page to working with hundreds of workplaces and women internationally, it's that you need support. I've been blessed to have many great people working with me along the way – delegation is a key part of the menopause journey. Concentrate on your areas of strength and delegate, if you can, those areas that are not your forte.

So tackle your symptoms as we talked about already, but when it comes to having your own business:

- Establish a routine – plan your day ahead.
- Don't be afraid to ask for help.
- Delegate, delegate, delegate some more – be honest with yourself and know your strengths and weaknesses.
- Have clear boundaries between work and home – if you work from home this can be tricky, but it warrants dedication, otherwise you may get burnt out and exacerbate your symptoms.
- Take your breaks.
- Have fun downtimes. When you're running your own business, you can get caught up in the excitement of growth, but you need time to replenish your own fuel tank. You need time for fun, for exercise, to be with your family and friends. Downtime will help you to be more productive and more passionate about your work.

WHAT I HAVE LEARNED FROM WORKPLACES

I'm still learning, and in every workplace I work with I learn something different. But one thing that continuously comes up is how relieved people feel when they have knowledge. This is reinforced by both men and women: it is key that this conversation is open and accessible to all people in the workplace. Closely tied to this are the smiles that I've seen, both on Zoom and in rooms, from both women and men when they can get together and understand they're not alone and feel supported by their employers and colleagues. Something beautiful happens when you bring people together and you share the subject of menopause – the relief, the laughter and the empowerment that helps people is second to none. A seed is sown and great things are building in many workplaces. Many have continued the work I have started by introducing internal support groups, menopause advocates and other supports. What I find most exciting and reassuring is how many workplaces are taking a long-term view of menopause and planning for it in their company structure.

TOP TIPS TO SUPPORT YOU DURING YOUR WORKING DAY

- Breathe: your breath is with you always and is a constant support in times of stress.
- Establish a morning routine.
- Avoid caffeine, especially before meetings, as it can trigger anxiety and your bladder.
- Be your own champion – listen to your body.
- Ditch perfectionism.
- Prioritise sleep at night.
- Take each day as it comes.
- Establish boundaries: these will be your best friend through these years, both inside work and outside, and they will protect your time, which is key.
- Get organised: use lists and whatever else can help you keep on top of your day.

- Technology is amazing: use any app that will support you.
- Delegate where possible.
- Preparation is the name of the game.
- Leave the white jeans at home.

Part 3: Your Options

14

Uncovering HRT

The area that I've received the most questions about over the last number of years is definitely HRT. It's a complex subject with a rollercoaster history behind it, very much in sync with the rollercoaster of hormonal havoc that can happen in menopause.

So what is HRT (also called HT or MHRT)? Simply put, it's adding hormones (oestrogen, progesterone and/or testosterone) that have declined in the body during and following the menopause years. But to understand it in more detail, we must start by looking at its history.

THE ROLLERCOASTER HISTORY OF HRT

The idea of adding hormones to the body didn't just come with the development of HRT. In AD 623 in China, San Si Miao was the first to document the use of organ extracts to treat disease. In the nineteenth century, the various forms of oestrogen were discovered, along with progesterone. Then in 1941/2, Premarin (oral HRT made from pregnant mares' urine) hit shelves in Canada and the US and soon became available worldwide. HRT was well and truly born.

The 1960s was the golden age of HRT. The advertising of the time (think Don Draper and *Mad Men*!) showed HRT as being glamorous, leading to endless youth. *Vogue* put HRT on the front cover when Dr Robert Wilson published his book *Feminine Forever* in 1966. He famously wrote that taking oestrogen would allow women to retain their femininity. We have moved far away from this kind of thinking today, but it did put menopause at centre stage.

In 1993, the Women's Health Initiative (WHI) and then, in 1996, the Million Women Study began. The WHI was the first randomised clinical trial to track the use of hormone therapy in healthy post-menopausal women. The study enrolled post-menopausal women aged fifty to seventy-nine and over a hundred thousand women were involved, covering many health aspects – twenty-seven thousand were involved in the HRT trial.

In 2002, the combined HRT aspect of the WHI study was stopped. It reported HRT to be a cause of breast cancer, stroke and heart attack. Overnight, women flushed their HRT down the toilets and abandoned all medications due to the media-raised fears.

In 2015, NICE (the National Institute for Health and Care Excellence in the UK), after reviewing data and safety concerns in relation to HRT, published guidelines that are now a global reference point for the prescription of and advice regarding HRT, and from 2018 onwards, menopause HRT use has increased again, as global awareness about the flaws in the previous studies gained momentum – ranging from the age of participants, existing underlying conditions and peri/menopausal symptoms being excluded, oral products being used and more. Newer, safer HRT options are constantly emerging and are frequent topics in the media.

NATURAL VERSUS SYNTHETIC

When I started to investigate HRT, I found a lot of the terminology confusing, and none more so than 'natural' and 'synthetic'. It's important to clear this up, as I think these words can be misleading.

A HRT product might be described as 'natural' because of the source it is made from – it may come from a plant (Mexican yam or soya) or animal (mares' urine). 'Natural' may also be applied to a product when its chemical structure is identical to that of oestrogen produced by the human body.

But natural, in my book, is when the human body produces hormones itself. So all forms of hormones not produced by the body are synthetic.

When products are described as 'bioidentical' this confusion becomes more apparent. There is an implication here (primarily due to marketing) that these are natural products and may be different from synthetic oestrogen. They are all synthetic.

The definition of synthetic is something made by combining chemical substances rather than being produced naturally by plants or animals. Thus any form not made by and spread throughout the human body is synthetic. The source may be a plant or animal or other, but it will still have gone through a process of chemical extraction and stabilisation. This is not to say synthetic is wrong – it is simply to understand the terms, and especially the marketing concepts, you may come across in your menopause journey.

Body identical versus bioidentical

These terms are often used in marketing material and really confuse the subject when they shouldn't. They also mean different things in different countries. It is important to understand what each means. You may hear 'plant-based hormones', 'body identical' and 'bioidentical' in the same sentence.

Body identical:

- Oestradiol via the skin (transdermal) or oral (e.g. Fematab or Qlaira).
- Made synthetically from yams.
- Molecularly the same as what your body produces.
- Considered the 'gold standard' starting regimen due to its safety profile.
- Regulated and controlled.
- Most standard forms of transdermal HRT prescribed by doctors are body identical.

Bioidentical:

- Another word for 'compounded hormones' – basically, a compounding pharmacy or clinic will make up a bioidentical mix of hormones that is individual to you, 'custom compounded'. The formulation may include oestrogen, testosterone, DHEA, thyroxine and melatonin.

- Can be made synthetically from yams or soya beans.
- Stated as a natural product – the main ingredient, oestradiol, is identical to that used in HRT.
- Molecularly, the oestrogen element is the same as what your body produces.
- Not regulated and no standard applies.
- Can be sold over the internet without a prescription – a common example is natural progesterone cream.
- Not endorsed by any menopause society globally.

THE HRT EQUATION

The backbone of HRT is replacing oestrogen, progesterone and sometimes testosterone. What your body may need is individual to you and will be dictated by the symptoms you are experiencing. To understand the HRT equation, and make the right decision for you, we need to go back to these three key hormones.

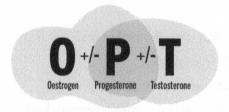

Oestrogen – the queen bee

Our bodies can produce four key forms of oestrogen, as discussed earlier. The most common form used with HRT is 17b oestradiol, which is body identical (sometimes called natural, as explained above). This means it has the same molecular structure as the oestradiol that our bodies produce.

Most transdermal HRT (delivered through the skin) is made from soya beans or yam extract. The conjugated equine oestrogens (CEE), made from pregnant mares' urine, contain oestrone sulphate, another oestrogen.

Progesterone – the protector (of the endometrium)

This calming, nurturing hormone plays a key role, as we saw earlier – it is the 'dancing partner' of oestrogen and responsible for so much in our bodies. It is essential if you have a womb, as it may protect you from endometrial hyperplasia (a build-up of endometrial tissue), which can in some cases lead to endometrial cancer. (In certain cases, progesterone may be prescribed where there is no uterus and a history of endometriosis.)

Progestogen is an umbrella term for both progesterone (the naturally occurring hormone in your body) and progestins, the synthetic versions which were created to protect the endometrial lining and also as a form of contraception. The most common form is micronised progesterone, which closely mirrors the progesterone our ovaries make in the second half of our menstrual cycle. Micronised refers to the very fine milling of the larger molecule which allows it to be absorbed better by the body.

You may see micronised progesterone or progestins like dydrogesterone, drospirenone and medroxyprogesterone acetate on your ingredient list.

Micronised progesterone:

- Has a safer breast/VTE (blood clot)/cardiac profile than synthetic progestogens
- Is taken via tablet at night and has a mild sedative effect so may help with sleep
- May not control bleeding as well as synthetic progestogens
- Is licensed for oral use only, but many menopause experts advise vaginal use to women who are sensitive to the effects of oral oestrogen

Progestins are similar to progesterone but not composed of the same molecular structure. They are often derived from testosterone and can therefore work on other receptors in the body as well as on progesterone, which can lead to side effects in some people.

The Mirena coil is an intrauterine device which is inserted into the uterus and releases a progestin. It:

• Protects the uterine lining
• Controls heavy bleeding (for most women)
• Is a contraceptive device
• Can be used as the progesterone part of the HRT equation

Remember, you can get pregnant in perimenopause so contraception is still required when needed. The Mirena coil contains the progestin levonorgestrel. Side effects of levonorgestrel may include acne, hair loss, mood changes and weight gain.

Progestins are not equal to progesterone, and many women may respond differently to the various forms of progestogens that may be used. If you are sensitive to the progestogen aspects of your HRT regime, generally they can reduce after one to two months – just keep track of what you are experiencing so you can discuss with your doctor.

Testosterone

Often thought of as the key male hormone, this is equally important for women. It can be helpful when oestrogen and progesterone settle down in the body, yet exhaustion, energy, libido and concentration are not improving. Its only clinical recommendation at the time of writing is for low libido. Testosterone is also known to strengthen bones and muscle mass. A blood test may be taken to assess testosterone levels before it is prescribed, but this is not always the case. It is applied transdermally, through a gel or cream.

In post-menopause, the average oestradiol level will have fallen by 80 per cent, and the average testosterone level by 25 per cent. If a person has experienced an oophorectomy (both ovaries taken out), the testosterone can fall between 40 and 50 per cent.

Randomised clinical trials of testosterone to date have not demonstrated the beneficial effects of testosterone therapy for cognition, mood, energy and musculoskeletal health.

WHICH ROAD DO YOU TAKE?

HRT can be complex, so the HRT roadmap here shows the high-level routes you can follow. Remember, the options you have will be determined by you and your doctor based on your current and past medical history.

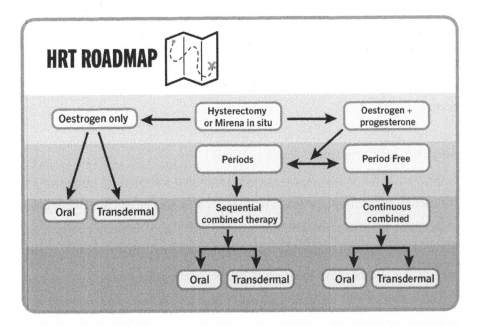

The first place to start is 1) whether you have had a hysterectomy or have a Mirena coil or 2) you have a uterus. This will determine whether you need oestrogen only or oestrogen and progesterone. Oestrogen can encourage the growth of the womb lining and lead to endometrial hyperplasia (a thickening of the womb lining), which may, in turn, lead to cancer of the endometrium (lining of the womb). To avoid this, progesterone is given with oestrogen.

HRT = O + P

If you have had a hysterectomy or have a Mirena coil, then progesterone may not be needed. The caveat to this is where a woman has a history of endometriosis and has had a hysterectomy – in this scenario, progesterone may also be required. This will be based on recommendations from your consultant.

HRT = O

When you have a uterus, the next step depends on whether you are still having periods or not, in which case you'll take sequential combined (cyclical) HRT if you're having periods or continuous combined HRT if you're not having periods.

Sequential combined (cyclical) HRT

Sequential HRT works in a sequence: oestrogen followed by progesterone. It's used in perimenopause when periods are still happening, whether regular or irregular. It is the most common form of HRT used in perimenopause, as the uterine lining can be thicker and irregular bleeding more common. Heavy periods can also be more common in the perimenopause years.

The sequence will be oestrogen daily (typically in transdermal form) and progesterone for ten to fourteen days monthly – the number of days depends on the type of progesterone used. An oral combination can also be used – a common market name is Trisquens. Generally, there is a monthly withdrawal bleed (85 per cent of women experience this), which is usually light.

Continuous combined HRT

This is often referred to as 'period-free HRT' – if your periods have stopped for more than a year, then continuous combined HRT may be offered.

You will take oestrogen and progesterone daily, via a tablet or transdermally. The Evorel Conti patch is a very common form where both hormones are released at the same time. It can also be transdermal oestrogen and nightly progesterone.

As your body gets used to it, you may experience spotting but this should settle down – if not, please talk to your GP.

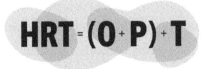

$$HRT = (O + P) + T$$

What about testosterone?

Many women do extremely well on oestrogen and progesterone once they find the form that suits them best and give it time to settle in the body. If after six months you are still experiencing loss of libido, tiredness and brain fog, then a conversation should be had with your GP to discuss adding testosterone to your HRT regime. (See Chapter 1 for more on testosterone.) As mentioned, under current guidelines testosterone is only medically prescribed for low libido.

Tibolone

This is not a pure form of HRT and is generally used for post-menopause. It is a synthetic hormone made from Mexican yam. When absorbed by the body, it is converted into substances that work similarly to oestrogen, progesterone and testosterone. As such, it works differently in different parts of the body. For example, in the brain it works like oestrogen and may prevent hot flushes from occurring. It mimics the protective aspect of oestrogen in the bones (but is not as strong a protector as oestradiol) and may also help with vaginal dryness. The progesterone aspect protects the uterine lining from an excess of growth, and the testosterone can help mood and libido. It is sometimes prescribed where there has been endometriosis and may also help with low libido.

It is only prescribed once periods have stopped for one year. It may be recommended to prevent bone loss but not for cardiovascular protection. As it may interfere with breast cancer therapies, it is contraindicated for use in women with breast cancer.

TYPES OF HRT

New forms of HRT are coming onto the market each year. The first step is understanding the various forms available and then seeing what form suits you best. We can break it into two main types – transdermal and oral. Within that, 'systemic' means the medication goes throughout the body, while 'local' means it impacts the local area where it is applied.

Transdermal forms of HRT are absorbed through the skin and replace hormones in your body in a way that closely mirrors how our ovaries produce them. They bypass the liver, hop straight into the blood vessels from the skin and then make their way around the body. Transdermal forms are now the first treatment option for those with risk factors, a history of deep-vein thrombosis or who are overweight.

Oral HRT has to be absorbed by the small intestine and broken down by the liver before it can make its way to the blood vessels.

Transdermal HRT

This comes in many forms, and each form has its own nuances and key tips for application.

Patch:

- Can be oestrogen only or a combined patch containing oestrogen and progesterone
- Gives a steady release of hormones over its duration of use
- Can be used for sequential or combined options

- Generally applied once or twice weekly
- Best applied to your bum, an easier place to remove it from and also you don't see it!
- Can be applied to the thigh, hip or lower abdomen also
- Vary where you put it – skin is sensitive, and if you apply to the same area of skin each time you may experience increased sensitivity

Gel:
- Oestrogen only or testosterone only
- Applied once or twice daily
- Best applied to your upper arm or thigh
- Don't rub it in – glide it onto your skin
- Allow it to dry before you get dressed
- Don't moisturise the area where you applied it

Spray:
- Oestrogen only
- Applied once or twice daily
- Best applied to your arms
- Allow it to dry before you get dressed
- Don't moisturise the area where you applied it

Local oestrogen (see Chapter 5 also):
- Pessary, cream or tablet – common types include Imvaggis, Ovestin, Vagirux, Vagifem, and Gina (used in post-menopause)
- Pessary containing oestriol 0.03mg
- Tablet, which dissolves in the vagina, contains 10mcg oestradiol
- General dose is nightly for two to three weeks and twice a week thereafter

Implant:
- Inserted under the skin into the abdomen
- Generally used where the symptoms are not responding to the regular forms of HRT

- Can include oestradiol (25–50mg), testosterone (100mg) or a combination
- Needs to be replaced every five to six months

Oral HRT

These are tablets which are taken daily and can be oestrogen only or oestrogen and progesterone (combined). Oral HRT tends to aggravate migraines for those who have a history of them, and poor absorption in the gut can be experienced by those who have IBD. If you are vegan, be aware that all oral oestrogen contains lactose. Oral HRT should be taken with food, with the exception of Utrogestan, which is best taken just before food – but this isn't always practical when taking at night.

HOW DO I DECIDE IF HRT IS FOR ME?

Making an informed choice is essential, so understanding the benefits and risks of HRT for your personal circumstances is the starting point.

The first thing to look at is your quality of life. If you know you are just not yourself and not enjoying life, then this may be the time to look at your HRT options. Your doctor will consider your symptoms, and whether they are mild, moderate or severe. You can also factor in the protective aspect of oestrogen for your bone and heart health.

The European Menopause and Andropause Society state that, for the majority of women, the benefits of HRT 'outweigh the risks, especially for symptomatic women before the age of 60 years or within 10 years after menopause'.

This ties in with what I have heard from hundreds of women for whom HRT has been a lifesaver. (Don't worry if HRT is not for you – I have you covered in Chapter 15.)

I never did well on the pill, so I was doubtful re HRT. My hot flushes were driving me mad. My doctor wanted me to try HRT. I was very reluctant as I thought it would be similar to the pill in how my body didn't like it, but I went with it. I used the smallest amount of gel and a few hours later I was in A&E. I had a blood clot. HRT is not for everyone, that's for sure.

– Josephine

RISKS OF HRT

As with every medication, HRT has its risks. The route of administration is important here in understanding these risks. Below are some of the potential risks you may have heard of.

Blood clots

This is also referred to as venous thromboembolism (VTE). If a blood clot happens in the legs, it is called a DVT (deep-vein thrombosis), if it is in the lungs it is a pulmonary embolism, and it may also happen in the brain.

There is a small increased risk of VTE with using oral HRT – a tablet form that has to be broken down by the liver. The liver is key within the body when it comes to blood clotting – if you experience a cut, your liver will make coagulation factors. These are proteins in your blood that help control bleeding and work together to form a blood clot.

In women aged fifty to fifty-nine, using oral HRT will result in two additional cases of VTE per thousand. This risk is highest in the first year and also where there is a family history of clotting. Smoking and obesity add a further risk.

This risk is reduced with transdermal options, which are absorbed through the skin and bypass the liver, reducing the issue of blood clotting. The British Menopause Society (BMS) advises that transdermal HRT should be considered for women at high risk of VTE and for those with a BMI over 30. A personal or family history of blood clotting does not preclude the use of transdermal HRT, but medical guidance will be given.

Breast cancer

Since the WHI study, further clinical research has occurred in the area of HRT and breast cancer, and we now know:

- There is a small increased risk with increased duration of use with some types of HRT.
- This is small in real numbers: about three to seven extra cases per thousand users at five years, according to NICE guidance and the British Menopause Society's consensus statement.
- The level of risk will change based on the type of HRT used:
  » It is most evident with synthetic progestogens.
  » Oestrogen-only HRT shows no increase/minimal increase – WHI actually showed a reduced risk.
  » Micronised progesterone and dydrogesterone showed no increase at five years via observational studies, but more data is required.
  » There is no increased risk with vaginal oestrogen.
  » The route of oestrogen administration does not impact on risk – it is the same for oral and transdermal.

Other factors that may cause an increased risk of breast cancer are:

- Alcohol consumption over two to three units per day
- Weight gain
- Having your first child after thirty years
- A diet high in saturated fats
- When natural menopause happens after the age of fifty-four

Facts are vital here. When we look at statistics, we know that excess weight and excess alcohol consumption pose a greater risk of breast cancer than HRT, as shown in the chart here, produced by the British Menopause Society. Bottom line: the risk of breast cancer caused by HRT is small and decreases once HRT is stopped.

When the HRT regimen is oestrogen with micronised progesterone,

Understanding the risks of breast cancer

Women's Health Concern

A comparison of lifestyle risk factors versus Hormone Replacement Therapy (HRT) treatment.

Difference in breast cancer incidence per 1,000 women aged 50-59.
Approximate number of women developing breast cancer over the next five years.

NICE Guideline, Menopause: Diagnosis and management November 2015

23 cases of breast cancer diagnosed in the UK general population

An additional four cases in women on combined hormone replacement therapy (HRT)

Four fewer cases in women on oestrogen only Hormone Replacement Therapy (HRT)

An additional four cases in women on combined hormonal contraceptives (the pill)

An additional five cases in women who drink 2 or more units of alcohol per day

Three additional cases in women who are current smokers

An additional 24 cases in women who are overweight or obese (BMI equal or greater than 30)

Seven fewer cases in women who take at least 2½ hours moderate exercise per week

Women's Health Concern

Women's Health Concern is the patient arm of the BMS.
We provide an independent service to advise, reassure and educate women
of all ages about their health, wellbeing and lifestyle concerns.

Go to **www.womens-health-concern.org**

BMS
British Menopause Society

March 2017

www.womens-health-concern.org
Reg Charity No: 279651
Company Reg No: 1432023

www.thebms.org.uk
Reg Charity No: 1015144
Company Reg No: 02759439

studies suggest no increased risk of breast cancer for five years. This is the safest HRT regimen to take in the long term. For oestrogen receptor negative breast cancer, HRT is not recommended currently as a first-line treatment. Limited studies (a meta-analysis by Poggio *et al.* in 2022) showed a small increased risk of recurrence for hormone negative breast cancer, which was less than that for hormone sensitive breast cancer and wasn't statistically significant. In essence, there currently isn't sufficient data. For oestrogen receptor positive breast cancer, HRT is not recommended currently.

Endometrial cancer

In the history of HRT development, progesterone was found to be important to protect the endometrial lining, so it was added to the equation alongside oestrogen where a woman had a uterus. This protects the uterus from endometrial cancer, as oestrogen is not left unchecked to encourage growth. Studies have shown that using a Mirena coil will decrease the chance of developing endometrial cancer by 20 per cent.

Ovarian cancer

Currently, there is conflicting data on the risk of ovarian cancer and HRT, with one meta-analysis showing the ovarian cancer rate increasing by 1 in 10,000 women, but this is not shown in other studies.

Stroke

According to the British Menopause Society's consensus statement on HRT in menopausal women, published in 2020, the literature assessing the risk of stroke with HRT shows that the risk of stroke is age related and low in women under sixty. Transdermal oestradiol may be considered for women over sixty or with risk factors. The type of progestogen used might also have an effect, so micronised progesterone or dydrogesterone should be considered with transdermal oestradiol for those at risk. There seems to be a small increase in the risk of stroke with oral oestradiol, which is probably related to dosage, so the lowest possible effective dose may be prescribed.

Colon cancer

Small studies have shown a possible reduction in the risk of colon cancer among recent post-menopausal HRT users for combined HRT only.

BENEFITS OF HRT

Once you find the HRT regimen that works for you, it may help to alleviate many or all of the symptoms you are experiencing. This will lead to improved quality of life and emotional balance, with the caveat that you also address any lifestyle factors. Some other benefits are as follows:

Heart health: Oestrogen receptors are found throughout the body, with many in the heart. Oestrogen protects the heart and also protects against high blood pressure, heart disease and bad cholesterol. The window of opportunity in relation to heart health is when HRT is started within ten years of menopause or under the age of sixty years. Transdermal options are again the preference here. HRT is not currently recommended as a prevention for cardiovascular disease.

Bone health: Numerous studies have noted the beneficial effect of HRT on bone health. HRT is not a first-line treatment for osteoporosis or osteopenia but can help in protecting bone health and can be an added bonus for women experiencing symptoms or early menopause.

Cognitive function: Anecdotally, women report improved memory and concentration when taking HRT. However, there are no completed clinical trials at this time to state that HRT will prevent dementia. Research in this area is currently being undertaken by Dr Lisa Mosconi to look at the impact of oestrogen on the female brain (see Chapter 8).

SIDE EFFECTS OF HRT

OESTROGEN	PROGESTOGENS
Bloating	Mood swings
Vaginal bleeding/spotting	Vaginal bleeding/spotting
Breast tenderness	PMS symptoms
Nausea/indigestion	Headaches
Fluid retention	Breast tenderness
Heartburn	Constipation/diarrhoea
Leg cramps	Acne
Headaches	Fluid retention

In many cases, the common side effects of HRT settle within the first few weeks and certainly within three to six months. If not, after six months it should be reviewed with your GP, discussing a possible change of type or dosage in the HRT you are taking. Irregular bleeding may be due to an imbalance in your dose and will need to be investigated by your GP.

Remember, HRT takes time to settle in your body and everyone will respond at a different rate and to the various routes of administration. If you find the side effects are creating an additional challenge, you have options to support you through this.

For many of the side effects of oestrogen, such as bloating, fluid retention or headaches, changing the route of administration or the dose may help. Discuss this with your doctor. For breast tenderness, evening primrose or starflower can be helpful. And if you're experiencing nausea or indigestion, try taking it with food to avoid this.

For the side effects of progesterone, such as mood swings and PMT symptoms, again, consider changing the route of administration. You might also consider changing the progestogen – you could be sensitive to the type, so changing from progesterone-derived to testosterone-derived or vice versa might help. If you are post-menopause, you can discuss with your doctor changing to continuous combined HRT or tibolone, as this can avoid the side effects that progesterone might bring.

FOLLOWING UP WITH YOUR GP

A review will be required, generally after three months, to see how you are responding to treatment. You should raise any side effects or complications and see if you need to tweak your dosage. If you are taking testosterone, ideally your levels should be checked within the first three months. If you see no improvement with taking testosterone after three to six months, it is a good idea to discuss stopping the medication with your doctor.

NON-HORMONAL MEDICAL OPTIONS

Not everyone can take HRT. Some contraindications can be:

- Abnormal vaginal bleeding
- Recent heart attack
- Recent blood clot in your legs or lungs
- Womb cancer
- Undergoing treatment for breast cancer
- Liver disease
- Uncontrolled high blood pressure
- Peanut allergy – for some types of HRT, not all

Family history is not a contraindication and requires medical review.

In some cases, based on personal medical history, HRT may not be an option (or the route of administration needs to be carefully considered). But other avenues, referred to as non-hormonal options, may be investigated.

Antidepressants

There is a history worldwide of the overprescribing of antidepressants in menopause, which makes this tricky territory. However, in some cases where

HRT is contraindicated, they can be of benefit in relieving some of the symptoms of menopause. Studies have found that SSRIs (selective serotonin reuptake inhibitors) not only helped with depression but also had an impact on the vasomotor symptoms of menopause – those systems aligned with our body's thermostat, the hot flushes and night sweats – because of their effect on serotonin, which plays its part in the thermostat-regulation process in the body. The doses required to help with menopause are generally lower than those used for depression. Just remember that antidepressants are not the first line of treatment for menopause, but can have an essential role to play either where HRT is contraindicated or where a person is experiencing depression. HRT can be taken with antidepressants.

Other medications

Gabapentin (Neurontin) is a medication used to treat various neurological disorders. For some women, it is effective in reducing hot flushes; it is particularly effective for night sweats if taken before bedtime. Side effects include dizziness, feeling drowsy, dry mouth, tiredness and weight gain.

Pregabalin, another neurological medicine, is commonly used for seizures, pain and fibromyalgia. It can help with the symptoms of anxiety in menopause and can be taken with tamoxifen and aromatase inhibitors. Its side effects are similar to gabapentin but less noticeable.

Clonidine (Dixarit) is a medication used for high blood pressure or migraine and can also help with hot flushes. Certain side effects have been noticed, including dry mouth, dizziness, constipation, difficulty sleeping and drowsiness.

Oxybutynin is used to treat an overactive bladder and can also help with hot flushes and night sweats. It can be taken with tamoxifen and aromatase inhibitor. Side effects may include diarrhoea, stomach cramps, dry eyes and mouth, headaches and nausea.

I went to my GP and told her I wanted HRT, and I haven't looked back since. I'm only sorry that I hadn't been given information on it fifteen years ago! I feel that things could have been very different for me. And now, so far so good. I feel my emotional state is more balanced. I'm sleeping way better. I'm in better form overall, and my sex life is slowly getting better. I think my atrophied cervix is recovering from years of discomfort. I'm retraining my brain not to kick into defence mode and allowing myself to relax and find pleasure instead of pain in our intimate life.

– Anon

HRT FAQS

What do I need to do before I can start HRT?

Your GP will do a full review of your general health – this may include bloods (to rule out any underlying conditions like thyroid), a weight check and a blood pressure check. Your GP needs to understand your symptoms and whether they are mild, moderate or severe. This will determine your possible treatment options. Ideally, the consultation should also discuss key lifestyle factors like alcohol intake, exercise, smoking and diet.

My best friend is doing great on HRT – I tried it and it didn't help me at all. Why?

The first thing to look at is the form of HRT you are using – each one can have different results for different people. If you have any issues with absorption from the bowel this may impact the amount of oestrogen that gets absorbed and sent throughout your body. You may need to look at a higher dose or change the transportation method. I would also encourage you to look at your lifestyle. Diet, exercise and sleep have a huge part to play and there may be an imbalance here to address.

When is the best time to start HRT?

It all goes back to the symptoms. How are you feeling? What symptoms are you experiencing, and what is their impact on your day-to-day life? You can start HRT while you are still having periods (sequential HRT, as discussed earlier). If your periods have stopped and you are post-menopause then you can discuss continuous combined HRT with your doctor. Tibolone might also be reviewed here as an option. The best time to start HRT is under the age of sixty and within ten years of menopause.

How long can I take HRT for? Is it only for five years?

When you are on HRT, you will be monitored by your GP. Throughout these years, the risks and benefits will be discussed and reviewed. As long as you are having this ongoing review, you can take HRT for as long as your doctor advises. You may come to a stage when you would like to take some time off HRT so you can assess where you are in relation to your symptoms. This will also allow you to know that you are benefiting from the medication. The key risk you may have heard of in taking it for more than five years is in relation to breast cancer – there is a small increased risk of breast cancer when you are fifty years old and taking it for over five years. But you have to look at that risk compared to alcohol consumption and weight too. The decision you take will be individual and personal. Once you are reviewing it with your doctor when you feel you need to, ideally on an ongoing basis, then you are in a position to make informed decisions throughout your years on HRT.

Can I start HRT after the age of sixty?

In theory, yes – however, we know starting HRT before the age of sixty offers higher benefits. Some studies suggest starting HRT after sixty may have a negative impact on cognitive function and won't be associated with a cardiovascular benefit.

How do I know I am on the right dose?

Your GP will start you on a low dose and work with you to monitor how your body responds to the new hormones it is absorbing. We know that often a low dose can work effectively for many symptoms of menopause. The aim is to get to a level where the symptoms are controlled and that may take time and patience. Many women do very well once they find their 'sweet spot' of oestrogen and progesterone. If after three to six months your symptoms remain unchanged then you may want to consider:

- The route of administration – maybe change from tablets to a transdermal form or vice versa
- A dosage increase
- Any other medications that may be interfering – for example, barbiturates (for anxiety, insomnia, seizures), carbamazepine or phenytoin (both for epilepsy and seizures)
- Ensuring the patch, if that's what you're using, is sticking properly to your skin
- Ensuring any other underlying condition has been ruled out – for example, thyroid disease, diabetes, chronic stress
- Discussing whether testosterone may help if just oestrogen and/or progesterone has been used to date
- How the symptoms you started with are now – HRT is not a cure-all for life's challenges and ills but should help to ease the symptoms you are experiencing

How do I know I am post-menopause?

Twelve months after your last period is defined as menopause. Everything after that is post-menopause. Your FSH blood result will also confirm that menopause has happened.

I am bleeding more heavily now and for longer than my normal period – is this right?

Irregular periods are very common in the perimenopause years. It is important to distinguish between small changes in your cycle and what might be termed abnormal uterine bleeding (AUB). This is where you bleed outside of your normal cycle and with greater duration, volume and frequency. This can be quite common due to the changes being created by your hormone levels, but it is important to have it checked out with your GP, as there can be many reasons for it – hyperplasia (build-up of the uterine lining), adenomyosis, polyps and so on. A transvaginal scan will be the starting point to check the status of the endometrium. This may be followed by a hysteroscopy if required.

I have started HRT and I am bleeding. Is this normal?

Yes! This is called breakthrough bleeding and can happen with oestrogen and progesterone therapy and also with oestrogen-only HRT. It should settle down after a few months but if not, please check with your GP. Very heavy ongoing bleeding should be checked immediately with your doctor.

Should all women take HRT?

Not all women will need HRT, but where it is required it plays a key role in a woman's quality of life. It is important to establish a good relationship with your doctor and ensure regular reviews so the risk–benefit balance is always being discussed. This will allow you to decide whether the benefits are outweighing the small risk (assuming transdermal is the regimen here).

Menopause often coincides with women's awareness of unhappiness in their family/relationship/work, etc., and menopause gets blamed. There is an expectation that HRT will make life 'happy' again. It is imperative that women who are unhappy at this stage in life make space to consider counselling or seek support to get perspective on their unhappiness, as often they need to set up boundaries for themselves that have been eroded by work or personal busyness (see Chapters 12 and 22 for more). Regardless of HRT, looking at your lifestyle is essential throughout your menopause years – establishing good habits here will set you up for success in the years ahead.

Do I need contraception when taking HRT?

HRT is not a form of contraception (with the exception of the halfway house which is the Mirena coil). In general, if you reach menopause under the age of fifty, you'll require contraception for two years after. If you reach menopause after fifty, contraception will be required for one year after.

* * *

My own opinion on HRT is that we don't want to reach a point where every woman is taking it as a matter of course. It may not be necessary for all women and may even be harmful in some cases. HRT should be an individual treatment with regular reviews to check how you are getting on, revisiting any risks and benefits as you age through these years. For many, the benefits gained from HRT will outweigh the small risks. Deciding to use HRT is your decision only: you just need to be aware of the facts so you can make an informed choice.

Remember that daily habits and lifestyle choices will greatly enhance your experience of menopause with no added risk. HRT is just another part of your toolkit.

We have one life and it is here to be lived. If you find your symptoms are interfering with everyday life, you must consider all options. If you are doing OK and maybe have just one or two symptoms that aren't causing you much trouble, then simply tweaking your personal toolkit might be the first step to take and making small changes to your daily lifestyle.

15

Other treatments

One key learning that is reinforced daily for me is that one size never fits all. This encompasses everything in life, and never more so than to the treatment options of menopause. I have seen it all: those thriving on HRT, those struggling on HRT, who just can't seem to get it to settle in their bodies, to those having great success with herbs and acupuncture. While data is still limited in many areas, I have seen first-hand the power of many of these therapies.

The most important thing is to listen to *you*: do what feels right for you and what you can see having a positive impact on your life.

What have I used to date? I think, by fifty-two, I had pretty much tried everything! I was introduced to homeopathy in London, fell in love with acupuncture in Dublin and discovered the healing power of herbs in Portmarnock. When my dad died, I received free counselling in college, and since then I have dipped back into talk therapy whenever I feel the need – it is one of the best things I have done on my menopause journey. So many things come up in these years, and sometimes it just helps to have an independent voice to chat to.

So let's look at some of the therapies that women have had success with in menopause.

HERBAL MEDICINE

Herbs have been used for healing for many thousands of years. It is estimated that 88 per cent of all countries use traditional medicine, such as herbal remedies, acupuncture, yoga, indigenous therapies and others. Many drugs (74 per cent) are, in fact, derived from plants.

Different parts of the plants can be used: flowers, fruit, leaves, seeds, roots and even small amounts of the bark of certain trees. In the right hands, herbs are natural, safe and can be effective. Herbs contain many phytochemicals and nutritive properties that can bring about a physiological, mental, emotional and even social benefit. Even just a few drops of the correct herb can have an almost instant effect – like echinacea for an infection or eucalyptus for a blocked nose. For chronic illnesses, where a lot of contributory factors are at play, a detailed consultation with a registered herbalist can provide the information for a personalised tonic, addressing all the health issues (see Resources).

You probably use herbs in everyday living without being aware – some turmeric or garlic, which have anti-inflammatory properties, in your soup at lunch, and rosemary or mint to aid digestion with your evening meal. You may use a few drops of lavender on your pillow at night to help you sleep, a rosemary shampoo to add shine to your hair or aloe vera lotion for sunburn. The following are some herbs you may find helpful with menopause symptoms:

- **Skullcap** supports people under stress, to help with overthinking and bring peace of mind.
- **Chamomile** aids sleep by cooling restlessness and agitation, both physical and mental.
- **Rosemary** may help with cognitive function by improving circulation to the brain but can raise blood pressure (so use in a tincture with caution).
- **Cayenne pepper** powder in tiny amounts supports circulation, effectively improving blood supply to all the vital organs.

- **Ashwagandha** (*Withania somnifera*) helps soothe your nerves by bringing down cortisol levels, and helps balance hormones.
- **Avena sativa,** made from oats, is another excellent herb for helping to calm the nerves yet it also improves energy. That's why horses are given oats: to calm them but make them run faster!
- ***Ginkgo biloba*** can also be used for cognitive function but cannot be used with some medications like Eltroxin, blood pressure medications or the pill.
- **Ginseng** also improves circulation to the brain but can increase heat in the body and blood pressure, so do not self-prescribe.

Always follow any precautions and instructions given with herbs. Some cannot be used in pregnancy, while breastfeeding or if on certain medications.

ACUPUNCTURE

The ancient practice of acupuncture originated in China approximately three thousand years ago. Treatment involves the insertion of very fine single-use sterile needles into specific points on the body to regulate the flow of 'Qi' (vital energy or life force) along pathways in the body known as meridians. Physical, emotional or mental imbalances obstruct the flow of Qi in the meridians or organs, leading to illness or pain. Acupuncture seeks to move the Qi within this system to rebalance and return to wellness. I used acupuncture every two weeks in my early perimenopause days to help with heavy periods. After three months I saw a dramatic positive change.

People often say 'no way' to me when they hear the mention of needles. I can tell you that the needles are so fine that most don't feel them being inserted. You may feel a mild tingle or dull ache as the acupuncturist adjusts the needle. Many people feel deeply relaxed during the treatment.

Your acupuncturist will take your medical history, read your pulse, look at your tongue and go through your symptoms to reach a treatment plan that focuses on your individual state of health and lifestyle. This informs them which point combinations are right for your whole body as well as your symptoms.

You can also have 'cupping' as part of your treatment. Another form of traditional Chinese medicine, cupping involves placing a bamboo, glass or plastic cup to the skin. Pressure in the cup is reduced by using a change in heat (fire cupping) or suctioning out air so the skin and superficial muscle layer is drawn into and held in the cup. This draws out toxins or congestion while drawing fresh blood and Qi to the area to improve circulation. It can be very relaxing too.

There are no contraindications to acupuncture, providing you are attending a trained practitioner. If you are pregnant or have a pacemaker, it is important to inform your practitioner. Some points are contraindicated in certain stages of pregnancy and some treatments (such as electro acupuncture) are contraindicated if the patient has a pacemaker. A trained practitioner will ensure a safe, individual treatment plan for each client.

> Acupuncture and herbs have been invaluable in my perimenopause. I always liked acupuncture but hadn't done it for many years. I found it a great support in my perimenopause, especially with helping me sleep better. I also love reflexology and that is a treat session for me – my body responds well to it. I had constipation in my early perimenopause years, and it always did the trick for me and got things back on track. It's so different for each of us – I think it's important women know there is so much out there to support them.
>
> – Jane

REFLEXOLOGY

Reflexology, which dates back to Ancient Egypt, is the practice of treating reflex points and locations on the hands and feet that correspond to different parts of the body. Energy pathways, or meridians, connect the feet to every organ and body part. These pathways become clogged or congested when our physical or emotional health is weakened, compromised or affected by sickness or stress. To assist the free flow of energy and return the body to its more natural state of health and well-being, reflexology can be employed extremely efficiently.

In menopause, reflexology works by helping to regulate the hormones and glandular functions of the body. Both the physical and emotional systems may benefit from it. It can assist in bringing the endocrine system back into balance by interacting with the hypothalamus and pituitary gland. In turn, this can lessen menopausal symptoms like hot flushes. Anxiety and stress levels can be decreased, as well as sleep problems, by soothing the central nervous system. Additionally, reflexology supports the uterus's natural health and suppleness by assisting the ovaries in controlling their oestrogen production. And last but not least, it can be of great benefit in preventing constipation and ensuring healthy bowel habits.

CBT

Cognitive behavioural therapy (CBT) can help you manage your behaviours by changing the way you think and behave. The North American Menopause Society (NAMS) recommends CBT as a step toward helping anxiety, stress, hot flushes, night sweats and sleep problems.

CBT is very useful in helping to understand and resolve anxiety. It systematically unpicks the process of anxiety – its beginnings, triggers, progression and play-out. Once that is all laid bare, it provides practical, useful everyday tactics to manage anxious thoughts.

What I like about CBT is the speed of effect. CBT gets to the point. It focuses on the present and future, not the past, and is very action-oriented. It is very down-to-earth and can deliver results within a short number of sessions.

There are plenty of self-help manuals and websites about CBT available, and the techniques can be applied to any area of your life. In relation to anxiety specifically, CBT is particularly effective. We know that anxious thinking leads to anxious feelings which results in anxious behaviour – CBT works by breaking the loop that leads to more anxious thinking and the vicious cycle of worry.

AROMATHERAPY

Aromatherapy is based on the idea that certain scents can have an impact on your psychological well-being. It includes the use of essential oils that can be applied to the skin or inhaled. Studies of aromatherapy suggest it may offer benefits in many areas, including anxiety, depression, digestive issues, sleep and pain management.

What I really like about essential oils is, first, that they are natural, derived from flowers, leaves, bark or roots of plants, and second, they act rapidly on the nervous system. A quick smell of an essential oil immediately triggers all fifty million smell receptors in your nose, which sends messages to your brain to help reduce your feelings of anxiety.

Choosing an essential oil is very personal, so play around and see what ones you like. I adore the tree essential oils (black spruce, Douglas fir, Atlas cedar) but others may prefer more citrus-based oils. As with anything, a good-quality essential oil is important – see Resources for details.

OTHER THERAPIES

Women I've talked to through work and my online community have had success with other therapies too, including:

- Bioenergy healing
- Homeopathy
- Kinesiology
- Lymphatic drainage
- Meditation and mindfulness

- Music therapy
- Osteopathy
- Reiki
- Somatic massage

* * *

These years are all about change. Your body is changing throughout, and that means that different approaches and strategies may all have a time and place in your personal journey. Being open to adapting your personal approach, your personal toolkit, is important, as is listening to your body and what it wants – this will help you to thrive through these years. This is your menopause, no one else's. Embrace the changes and adapt your approach throughout these years as needed.

Exploring supplements

Many people dislike certain foods or tastes, and this can reduce essential nutrient groups from their diet. For me, it is always food first – this is the best source of nutrition. But that doesn't work for everyone or in all cases. Your body may require higher doses of certain nutrients and vitamins than you can obtain from food – for example, vitamin D.

In this chapter, we'll explore supplements that can offer support during menopause. Be patient in looking for improvements, as it can take time for the body to absorb and reap the benefits of the nutrients contained within.

Be careful to follow dosage guidelines as indicated on product labels or based on guidance from your pharmacist or health-care professional.

I now had my box for all things menopause or perimenopause. Each part had to earn its spot from a therapeutic and safety/health perspective. I supplemented my box with acupuncture, reflexology and meditation, then signed up for Catherine's 'Thrive through Menopause' weekly sessions on Zoom.

So, what went into my box?

– My low dose of oral HRT (combined 1/10mg) – a month's supply

– Some good quality iron tablets

– My magnesium glycinate capsules

– My valerian drops (I need them less and less)

– Some herbal teas

– My candle and safety matches

– A little container of bath salts for my foot spa

– Essential oil with blending oil for a massage after the foot spa

– A good multivitamin, with B complex and D3

My mantra is a deep inhale and slow exhale, and to tell myself, 'There will be hard days but they will pass, so look forward to the good days.'

– Ciara

OMEGA-3

The brain is made up of 60 per cent fat. Fat is a vital component of a healthy and calm mind and body. Of all the oils, Omega-3 is the sacred one, the one that makes your body thrive. This brain-boosting nutrient provides anti-inflammatory benefits, not only to the brain but also to the heart. Omega-6 and -9 are more common in modern diets; omega-3 requires planning to ensure you have adequate levels.

Food sources include fish like salmon, mackerel, anchovies, sardines and herring. If you're feeling flush, a dollop of caviar gives a great boost of omega-3! And if you're not a fan of fish, there are other good food sources: flaxseeds, chia seeds, hemp seeds, olives, walnuts, almonds, avocados and soybeans.

If those food sources won't work for you, I would recommend using a supplement. When looking for a good supplement, look at the omega-3 levels of EPA and DHA. EPA is the portion responsible for making neurotransmitters, and DHA is responsible for cell building throughout the body. A daily intake of 250mg of EPA and DHA is recommended for the beneficial effect.

VITAMINS

B vitamins

The B vitamins play a vital role in maintaining a healthy nervous system, and they are an essential vitamin group in menopause, as our need for them increases as we age. This is because absorption declines due to digestive issues, and vitamin B12, in particular, is impacted by this change. Low levels may affect your cognitive function, bone mineral density and heart health, and your ability to manage stress.

While our bodies change in perimenopause, our dietary needs also change – nutrition can make the biggest difference at this time. Ensure you top up with a diet rich in B vitamins, and add plenty of fish, eggs, nuts and seeds to your diet.

There are several B vitamins and they all play a vital role in maintaining health during these years. They are necessary for strong adrenal glands, a healthy nervous system and the conversion of carbohydrates into the glucose we need for energy.

- **B2 (riboflavin)** is key for the release and activity of many hormones, including oestrogen. It also helps keep skin, nails and hair healthy. Good sources are milk and eggs.

- **B3 (niacin)**, along with B9, helps our bodies metabolise oestrogen and other sex hormones. It reduces blood cholesterol, dilates blood vessels and is often used as a supplement to prevent premenstrual headaches. It can also help with confusion, insomnia, memory loss, irritability and mood. If you're using B vitamins to help prevent hot flushes, be sure to use the form of niacin called niacinamide. Other forms of niacin dilate the blood vessels, which can worsen hot flushes, rather than relieve them – something we do not want!

- **B6 (pyridoxine)** is the hormone-regulating B vitamin and is a natural diuretic. When you get bloating before or during your period, this is when you may need B6. It may also help to promote calm moods and restful sleep. It interacts with oestrogen in the body. This vitamin is found in most foods and deficiencies are rare.

- **B7 (biotin)** is well known for its positive impact on hair, nails and skin. It can also keep mucous membranes healthy.

- **B9 (folic acid)** helps the body make and use oestrogen. It helps reduce forgetfulness, provides neuroprotection, eases irritability, can help insomnia and promotes the growth of healthy red blood cells (which is why a deficiency of this vitamin can lead to anaemia). Sources of folic acid include green leafy vegetables, nuts, beans and peas.

- **B12 (cobalamin)** is exceptional in many ways. While many vitamins and minerals are at work in your body to convert the food you eat into energy and keep things going smoothly, you will probably get the right dose of them by eating a well-balanced diet. The exception is B12. This vitamin is the key to unlocking the energy from the food you eat while keeping your nerves and blood cells healthy. As one of the most important B vitamins, it may help decrease mood swings, eliminate fatigue and prevent anaemia (low iron). Vegetarian sources containing high amounts of B12 include seaweeds, such as arame, wakame and nori; my favourites, fermented foods – pickles, sauerkraut, tempeh, tamari and miso; and finally, B12-enriched soy products. Animal-derived sources include eggs, milk and fish. You can also get food supplements rich in B12, which are blue-green algae, chlorella, barley green and spirulina.

Vitamin C

Our adrenal glands are in charge of the two key anxiety/stress hormones: cortisol and adrenaline. Vitamin C is water soluble and, while it is not stored in the body, it does accumulate in certain fluids and organs – some of the largest amounts accumulate in the adrenals. When we are under stress, we use our vitamin C up in record time. As our bodies do not produce vitamin C, we need to get it through our diet, so to ensure optimum health throughout our bodies, it is important to eat foods rich in this vital vitamin. Vitamin C is always my go-to at the first signs of a cold. Load up on the vitamin C foods listed below, and if you have an infection, then topping up with a vitamin C supplement might help. A higher dose taken over a few days may dramatically reduce the duration of a cold.

You may also come across liposomal vitamin C. This form contains the normal vitamin C but within two layers of phospholipids, allowing the vitamin C to be protected from gastric acid and enzymes and be absorbed more efficiently from the gut into the bloodstream.

Camu camu, a berry rich in vitamin C, is another excellent form, also providing B vitamins, potassium and many other minerals and vitamins.

Foods rich in vitamin C include citrus fruits, berries, goji berries, kiwis, tomatoes, apricots, peppers, broccoli, brussels sprouts and sweet potatoes.

Vitamin D – the sunshine vitamin

This could well be called the mood vitamin, in my view: it is one of the key vitamins needed by the body to keep us balanced. As we get older, our body's ability to absorb vitamin D reduces, which may cause a reduction in our ability to assimilate calcium. This may lead to an increased risk of osteoporosis, most especially in menopause. Vitamin D has a close relationship with calcium, both impacting the brain activity involved in neurotransmitter processing and the health of the adrenal and pituitary glands. Vitamin D helps the absorption of calcium, so it is worthwhile ensuring a diet rich in both.

For years we have associated vitamin D with stronger bones and teeth, but we now know it plays a key role in the immune system and mood. A lack of vitamin D diminishes the body's ability to produce feel-good brain chemicals, including serotonin and dopamine, so it is an essential aid in supporting mood.

We can get vitamin D from food sources but we are only able to take a very small amount this way. The main food sources are eggs, oily fish, cod liver oil, shiitake and button mushrooms and red meat. We can also get vitamin

D from sunlight on our skin (don't forget to wear SPF, especially if you burn easily). As a supplement, I prefer an oral-spray form of vitamin D – as it is an oil-soluble vitamin, there can be challenges in absorbing it, which makes the spray form more effective, with rapid absorption into the bloodstream.

When next having a blood test, it is worth getting your vitamin D levels checked, as most people these days are deficient in this vital vitamin.

MINERALS

Calcium
See Chapter 7.

Magnesium
Magnesium is a multitasker and plays a part in many processes in the body, from normal muscle function to bone health. It can help us relax; it is a key nutrient for the adrenal glands. When we are under stress, we actually lose magnesium. Food sources include:

- Wholegrain brown rice
- Avocado (one gives you 15 per cent of your daily required magnesium)
- Pumpkin seeds – 30g gives a whopping 317mg of magnesium, about 100 per cent of your recommended daily intake!
- Beans
- Nuts
- Dark leafy green vegetables like kale and spinach
- Quinoa
- Oats
- Raw cacao powder

What is magnesium? Magnesium is a mineral, one of the nineteen minerals considered essential for life and the fourth commonest mineral in the body. Most of the magnesium in our bodies is in our bones and teeth (roughly

60–65 per cent), the balance in the rest of the body and our blood (though our blood only houses 1–2 per cent). Magnesium is mostly utilised in the heart and brain, which may explain why it is so important for the nervous system and sleep. Interestingly, many of the symptoms of magnesium deficiency tick the box of menopausal symptoms, making it essential for your toolkit at this stage. Dr Carolyn Dean, author of the *Magnesium Miracle*, calls magnesium 'the spark of life'.

How does magnesium help? It is essential in your diet at all stages of life for everyone – from children, growing teenagers and active sportspeople to those in perimenopause and beyond. It plays a vital role in heart health (blood pressure and steady heartbeat), bone health, immune function, muscle function, brain health and energy transmission throughout the body. The main conditions helped by magnesium are asthma, fibromyalgia, migraines, headaches, night sweats, heart palpitations, osteoporosis, PMT, low mood, diabetes, aches, pains and inflammation.

Why are we not getting as much magnesium as we need? Many factors influence how much magnesium we absorb into our bodies. Alcohol and caffeine can impact absorption because of their diuretic effect. If you're exercising a lot, excess sweating will lead to loss of magnesium, and your muscles use more magnesium when you're active. How food is processed and cooked can decrease magnesium levels – for example, take white flour: magnesium is stored in the bran and the germ, which is lost in the milling process of the whole grains. Sugar also drains magnesium – for every molecule of sugar you eat, it takes fifty-four molecules of magnesium for your body to process it. Certain medications like acid blockers, antibiotics and diuretics can reduce absorption. If you experience a bout of vomiting, diarrhoea or urinary infection, this will result in a loss of magnesium. Those who are coeliac or have low stomach acid can't absorb magnesium as effectively from food as others. Finally, chronic stress impacts our gut health, which will inhibit the absorption and action of magnesium.

How do I know I am deficient? Many of the symptoms of low magnesium are similar to perimenopause symptoms – the commonest signs are:

- Cramps – you may experience more cramps, especially during your period.
- Restless legs – muscle twitches can be due to low magnesium, potassium, calcium and iron.
- Constipation – a very common sign of deficiency. Some forms of magnesium draw water to the bowel to help soften the stool. In addition, magnesium can help relax the intestines to allow the stool to move through.
- Brain fog – magnesium is needed for neurotransmitter function.
- Stress – our body uses up magnesium faster when stressed, and when we are low in magnesium we have a harder time handling stress, creating a vicious cycle.
- Palpitations – magnesium is essential for cardiac function.
- Calcium build-up in your muscles and tendons (calcific tendonitis) – this is very common in the upper arm and shoulder.
- Excess sweating – you will lose magnesium through night sweats and hot flushes, as well as vigorous exercise.
- Bloating – where there is low stomach acid, magnesium cannot be absorbed properly.
- Dental issues – frequent cavities can be a sign of low levels.
- High blood pressure, migraines, headaches, sleep issues, appetite loss and nausea may also indicate deficiency.

How should I take magnesium? Magnesium supplements come in many forms. The most effective are:

- Magnesium citrate: widely available and has a good absorption rate into the body. Initially, it may cause loose bowels so build up your intake slowly. The powder form (ionic magnesium citrate) is very well absorbed – it enters the cells throughout your body quickly and effectively. Dissolving in water also enhances absorption in the gut.

- Magnesium glycinate: also called magnesium bisglycinate – magnesium compounded with glycinate, an amino acid best known for its calming effect. The glycine molecule also reduces the impact of substances that might hinder absorption. It is often used for pain, anxiety, insomnia and tight muscles. It may help balance moods, calm the body and help the detoxification process.
- Magnesium taurate: taurine is an amino acid that is good for the heart, eyes, muscles and brain function.
- Magnesium aspartate: this form is good for fatigue.
- Magnesium malate: energising, best suited for those experiencing fibromyalgia.
- Magnesium orotate: a less common form, used for high blood pressure, angina, overall heart health and athletic performance.
- Magnesium threonate: this is magnesium that crosses the blood–brain barrier. It is the best form for its impact on long- and short-term memory.

You can incorporate magnesium flake baths and the use of magnesium body oil into your daily habits. A warm Epsom salt bath at the end of the day will relax your muscles and ensure a deep night's sleep too. Most people report the best effect is by taking magnesium at night-time just before bed.

> It took me some time to get to the bottom of what was going on with me, but when I looked at the symptoms of magnesium deficiency, I was literally ticking them all off. When I started eating more magnesium-rich foods and taking a supplement, it was like a shadow was lifted off me and I became myself again.
>
> – Siobhán

Zinc – unsung superhero of the immune system

Your immune system cannot operate at peak performance if you lack zinc. Over two hundred chemical reactions in our bodies need zinc to perform effectively. It is an important disease fighter and a protector of our immune system. It encourages our production of immune cells, giving us a better defence against viruses, and is known for its ability to help with respiratory-tract infections. Our ability to absorb zinc declines as we get older. If you don't have enough zinc in your body and infection hits, then inflammation can spread to other parts of your body.

Zinc-rich foods include pumpkin seeds, nuts, egg yolks, cheese, fortified foods, whole grains and seafood, especially oysters.

HERBAL SUPPLEMENTS

Adaptogens are herbs and plants that can help our bodies adapt to and handle stress in our environment and rebalance our hormones. They can help our bodies recover from short- and long-term mental or physical stress. Some have additional properties that may boost cardiovascular health, immunity, mood, cognitive issues and fatigue. Their effects can be far-reaching. (See Chapter 15 for more.)

Evening primrose oil

Many women take evening primrose oil to alleviate the symptoms of menopause. It helps with breast tenderness, and many women report it also helps with hot flushes.

Maca root

This has been used for thousands of years to lower the effects of stress and ageing on the body by decreasing cortisol levels. Maca is a great addition to the perimenopause diet. It is good for the adrenal glands, so may help with stress management. Maca may also help to balance your hormones due to its impact on the pituitary gland and the hypothalamus. Many women find it helps with hot flushes, night sweats, sleep issues, low mood and loss of libido. There are many forms on the market – Peruvian maca is the one I'd recommend.

Rhodiola

This enhances physical and mental performance, may help with low mood and improves sleep by altering the levels of dopamine, norepinephrine and serotonin in the brain.

Lemon balm

Otherwise known as *Melissa officinalis*, this herb enhances your memory. It is part of the mint family and is considered to be a calming herb, as it helps to reduce cortisol. Lemon balm has been used for many centuries to reduce stress, improve appetite and even ease pain and discomfort. It can be taken as a tea or in tablet form.

Passionflower

This can help relieve anxiety and insomnia, making it very useful in menopause. Research indicates it can boost the level of GABA in the brain, which calms brain activity, which may help you relax and sleep better.

Gotu Kola

This has been around for centuries and has been traditionally used to help alleviate anxiety, mental fatigue, low mood, memory loss and insomnia.

Magnolia

Traditional Chinese medicine has used this bark for years to help with anxiety, stress and sleep disturbances. A 2011 Italian contolled study compared the effectiveness of magnolia bark to soy isoflavones for mood disorders in menopause. The study found that the soy isoflavones did help the typical menopause symptoms of hot flushes, while the magnolia helped ease anxiety.

Black cohosh

This was originally used by Native Americans to help relieve period and labour pains. It has an impact on the serotonin levels in the body, which may have a knock-on impact on mood and hot flushes. It should be avoided if you have liver disease.

Sage

This is one of the easiest herbs to grow in your garden. I often just use the leaves to make tea. Research is ongoing into sage, which has an affinity for relieving hot flushes. You can take it as a tea or a herbal extract. Avoid if taking tamoxifen or blood pressure medication.

Saffron extract

Clinical trials have shown this to have a positive impact on mood. Saffron components work on serotonin production in the gut, where an estimated 90 per cent of this hormone is produced, hence the impact on mood.

AMINO ACIDS

Taurine

This non-essential amino acid (our body can make it using other essential amino acids) is a key part of the neurotransmitters in the brain. It is linked with cognitive function, learning, memory and mood, and may help to manage stress and promote good heart health. Food sources include shellfish, such as scallops, clams and mussels, and dark turkey and chicken meat.

L-theanine

Its big job is calming the key neurotransmitters like serotonin, GABA and dopamine. As such, it can be calming and relaxing. It is often given to help with sleep – not because it makes you sleepy, but due to the calming influence it has. It can reduce blood pressure, so please speak with your GP if you are on blood pressure medication. Food sources include green tea, black tea and some mushrooms (for example, *Boletus badius*).

5-HTP

Your body naturally manufactures the amino acid 5-hydroxytryptophan (5-HTP), which is used by your body to make serotonin. Depression, anxiety, sleep issues, weight gain and other health issues are all linked to low serotonin levels. 5-HTP is made from an African plant and may help with sleep and low mood. This should not be taken with antidepressants or St John's Wort.

FLOWER ESSENCES

Australian Bush flower essences and Bach flower essences are handy resources to have in your menopause toolkit, whether it's the emergency spray or rescue remedy.

- Emergency Essence – a mix of seven essences, which works like Bach Rescue Remedy but on different areas of the body and mind.
- Calm & Clear – my personal favourite. This combination helps us to slow down, take stock, replenish our minds and let go of unwanted worries – crucial in a world that is becoming faster and on the go 24/7.
- Women Essence – combines some key essences that have an affinity with female hormones, encompassing worry, hot flushes, fear, adrenal support and anxiety.

HOW TO READ A SUPPLEMENT LABEL

I am really picky about my supplements. I get annoyed when I see marketing ploys and evasive labelling that set products up to be something they are not. Take the time to read your labels: knowledge is power.

- Some forms of nutrients are more absorbable than others. Talk to the health-shop staff or a nutritionist if you are unsure of the form.
- Check when is best to take your supplement. Some supplements may work better when taken with food or at the start of the day.
- Look at the ingredient levels and the nutritional table or supplement facts

panel on the box to see how they compare to the recommended daily intake for that ingredient.

- See how much you need to take each day for best results. The value for money may not seem so good when you look at the dosage.
- Look for a supplement that combines ingredients, rather than buying them separately – this can increase your likelihood of taking it and reduce cost too!
- Excipients or fillers are sometimes used to bind active ingredients in tablet form. Try to find a source with minimal fillers.

* * *

The world of supplements is big business and evolving by the day. Knowing what you are putting into your body and understanding how it may benefit you is fundamental. A high-quality supplement with the right ingredients combined with a healthy lifestyle can support your optimum health, but where possible, food should be your primary source.

Part 4:
The 6 Ms of
Menopause

17

MOT – your menopause check-in

Having a tribe is an integral part of your menopause years. This will be your family, friends and work colleagues, but may also include your GP, women's health physiotherapist, pharmacist, therapist and health-shop advisor. Some you will interact with more regularly than others, but one essential aspect is the role of your GP.

THE GP VISIT

Many women tell me that they don't regularly have a check-up with their GP. For me, it is all about being empowered and in control of your health – your body. No one knows and understands your body as well as you do. Ideally, visit your GP on an annual basis from the age of forty-plus. This will allow you to stay on top of your health and be proactive in monitoring any possible conditions that might arise. A good check-in point is your birthday.

This is an important step and stands apart from perimenopause, as I believe it's a good thing to be in the habit of doing. Menopause does not always require medical treatment but a regular check-up keeps you ship-shape.

Sadly, although many voices are working to improve the situation, we also know that medical gaslighting exists in the form of a lack of concern and awareness in relation to women's health. I have heard many stories of appointments with doctors where women have been passed off, unheard, ignored and told to 'get on with it'. This is not acceptable, so don't be afraid to change doctor if you need to: have the confidence and empower yourself to find the support you deserve for your menopause years.

Booking your appointment

When you make your appointment, mention that it might be longer than usual because you want to discuss your menopause. A ten-minute appointment will not suffice – you will need more time, especially for your first appointment.

Your questions

When you attend your GP, be ready with your questions and be clear about what you would like to achieve in the appointment. The role of the doctor is changing, and will continue to change, to a more collaborative relationship overseeing your optimum health.

Print off a symptom checker (see Resources) and bring this with you. If you are experiencing brain fog, chances are you might forget some of the symptoms you are experiencing. This will also give you an idea, before you go to the appointment, of what may be menopause-related and what is not.

A copy of the NICE guidelines (evidence-based recommendations for health and care in England) for menopause might be helpful to bring too. As of October 2022, Irish doctors have access to a menopause quick reference guide, which outlines key aspects of treatment during these years.

List of medications, supplements and/or herbs

Have a written list ready of what you are taking that you can review with your doctor to ensure no contraindications exist with any possible prescriptions.

Be respectful of each other

GPs are not experts in all aspects of our health – they look after everyone, from babies to geriatric patients. Menopause is but one chapter in our lives, and they unfortunately receive very little training in this. You will have your personal views and so will your doctor. Ideally, there will be common ground, but if there isn't, this is where you need to be assertive and confident in the knowledge you have gained to ensure you get the support you need. This is your body and your health, and as such you need to be an empowered participant in the equation. Don't be afraid to say no when you're not in agreement, and make sure you get through all your questions.

Bring back-up

Your head may be in a spin, there may be information overload, or you might forget what you want to ask (a good reason to have that list ready!) Having your husband, partner or a friend with you can be a great help and can also help you feel more secure and less anxious.

The appointment

When you meet with your GP, several investigations may be discussed or taken, either at your first visit or on follow-up visits. Below are some procedures that may be required over these years, or specialists you might be referred to, with the essential starting point being your chat about the symptoms you are experiencing and how you are feeling.

Blood tests: I love nothing better than reading a blood test result – it so often gives me that Hercule Poirot moment! Blood tests can be a great indicator of how your body is doing. Some key ones are:

- CA-125 (this is used to test for early signs of ovarian cancer in people at high risk – your GP will determine if it is necessary)
- Cholesterol
- Coeliac disease
- Fasting insulin or HbA1c

- Iron
- Thyroid
- Vitamin D
- Vitamin B12
- White blood cell count

It's a good habit, too, to ask for a copy of the results so you can monitor them yourself. If you have been diagnosed with POI, an extended set of tests would be required.

Physical vaginal exam: You mightn't want to hear this, but this is another good way to keep on top of your vaginal health. Your doctor or a women's health physiotherapist will be able to assess the health of your vaginal tissues and alert you to anything that needs attention. A few minutes of discomfort could change your health outlook months and years down the line.

Contraception: Remember, you can get pregnant as you go through perimenopause, so you may want to discuss and consider your options with your GP.

Blood pressure: Regular blood pressure checks are essential.

Cervical smear: OK, no one gets excited about these, but they are very important, so make sure you keep on track and have one regularly. If you find them painful, a great tip is to apply an internal vaginal moisturiser – start the week before for a few nights and stop two nights prior to your smear. This may reduce discomfort, especially if you are experiencing vaginal dryness.

Breast check: Ideally, this is a check you'd do at home once a month – a nice habit is the first day of every month. It is good to check with your GP that you are doing it correctly.

DXA scan: Personally, I would like to see all women having access to a free DXA scan from age forty-five, at a minimum. Knowing your bone health (see Chapter 7) is crucial to protect and future-proof yourself. Your GP can refer you for a DXA scan.

Bowel scan: Currently, the National Bowel Screening Programme offers free bowel screening to people aged sixty to sixty-nine every two years. Bowel screening aims to detect signs of bowel cancer at an early stage, where there are no symptoms. If you have symptoms, you may want to discuss this with your doctor sooner.

HRT: As outlined in Chapter 14, it is important to understand your options based on your personal medical history when it comes to HRT. Ask your doctor:

- Why this regimen is being suggested and what exactly it is
- What are the benefits and risks, personal to you
- If you are starting on the lowest dose
- What are the common side effects to be aware of
- How often you will be checked once you start your HRT regimen
- For guidelines on how to apply it, if it's transdermal
- When you are to take it, if it's oral (remember, progesterone is best taken at night)
- How long you will be on HRT for
- If the suggested HRT will interfere with any other supplements or herbs you may be taking
- How often you should come for check-ups when on HRT
- What health and lifestyle suggestions they have for you

DERMATOLOGIST – MELANOMA

Skin cancer is extremely common, and it is another area where that window of opportunity that menopause offers us can help – we can be proactive and have our skin checked for any suspicious changes. This should be done on an annual basis from age fifty. Your doctor can refer you.

WOMEN'S HEALTH PHYSIOTHERAPIST

As outlined in Chapter 5, this will be your new best friend. Make this visit part of your annual, or even more regular, check-in on your health.

* * *

Currently, there are four complex menopause clinics in Ireland to which you can be referred by your GP. There are also several menopause specialist doctors/private clinics. Ideally, your starting point will be your local GP.

Making time for all these checks and taking control of your health is building the foundations of thriving through menopause and will empower you in your journey to future-proof your optimum health.

18

Movement – the essential step

Your body loves the feeling it gets from movement; it loves the stimulus it creates throughout your body. We need change in how we move throughout our lives, and never more so than in these years, when we can use movement to future-proof our bone, heart and brain health. We all know that making movement and physical activity part of our everyday lives can make an enormous difference to our overall health and well-being.

The benefits of movement and exercise are well documented and include:

- Weight management
- Management of blood sugar and insulin levels, lowering the risk of type 2 diabetes
- Lower blood cholesterol levels
- Lower blood pressure
- Enhanced cardiovascular health
- Strengthened bones and muscles
- Enhanced immune system
- Improved sleep
- Optimal brain health
- Improved mental health with endorphin release (the natural antidepressants)

Movement also burns off the stress hormone adrenaline. The very nature of movement helps every aspect of health, from building immunity to reducing everyday stress. While you are exercising, you are breathing more deeply and your mind is taken off any anxious thoughts; it helps you sleep better at night and releases those feel-good chemicals (endorphins) that are imperative for supporting balanced mood and reducing stress. Feel-good hormones will outrun stress hormones every time, and managing stress is one of the cornerstones of thriving through menopause.

As for the risks, once you have confirmed with your doctor that you're ready to go, there is no downside to moving daily.

WHY YOU SHOULD MOVE EVERY DAY

If we look back at our ancestors, life was full of constant activity, from hunting to basic survival. Humans thrive on movement – like animals, we are not built to lead sedentary lives.

Daily movement has much to offer us, but in today's world, it takes commitment and planning. I block out my exercise sessions in my calendar every week so I am fully committed to these times – they are non-negotiable. Yes, some weeks life gets in the way, but being committed to long-term movement is one of the best steps you can take for yourself for today and for the years ahead.

As we get older, our mobility and flexibility change, and this can also bring joint pain as you go through menopause. You want to stay mobile, limber and agile. This is where movement comes in. We also want to keep our bones and muscles strong, which means strengthening exercises.

Don't be hard on yourself

Keep reminding yourself of the benefits of movement, but at the same time, be kind to yourself. If you're new to exercise, it will take time. I was never athletic as a child and only discovered my love of running when I was forty-four (just at the start of my perimenopause). You can introduce movement into your life at any age, and it's important to keep it balanced. You will have days when your body is tired and that's OK. Life is busy, and we have many commitments and responsibilities in work, life and menopause. While I believe women are amazing, we don't have to be superwomen. Just listen to your body: it will tell you when it needs to rest and when you need to take things easier. Remember, you are in it for the long haul. Movement in your life is a marathon, not a sprint.

Mood and movement

I owe my love of walking in the mountains to my dad. We had many beautiful spots to walk through with the dogs when I was growing up, and I loved nothing more than heading out in the evenings for a walk in the forest. The sound of wind in the trees, the birds and the lovely chats we used to have are precious memories. So, however you move, just enjoy it and the mood boost you gain from the endorphins. We are lucky to be alive, and we are so lucky to be able to move, in whatever form this takes – it is something we should never take for granted.

When you are outdoors, remember to be present, enjoy the fresh air, and enjoy the sights and sounds of nature. Listen to the birds, to the leaves rustling in the trees and to the water flowing.

> The people I run with, the friendships and the laughter are what keep me going. I know, of course, there are many health benefits for my body and mind, but the laughter is the best thing. Running outdoors is just amazing – listening to nature, the sounds of water, looking around and taking the world in is what I love. When I trained for the marathon I kept my running group in constant states of laughter, getting pictured with firemen, gardaí and rugby players. Laughter is just so important!
>
> – Colette

TIPS FOR ADDING MOVEMENT TO YOUR LIFE

Create a movement mindset: Keep reminding yourself of all the health benefits you gain every time you move and this will encourage you, even on those occasions when Netflix and the couch appear more seductive. Remind yourself how great you feel after a movement session.

Make it easy: Arrange to go with a friend; keep your runners by the door; have your weights in the kitchen. If it's easy, there is a higher chance you will follow through!

Block the time in your calendar: It's more likely to happen if you have the time scheduled and allotted to your movement routine.

Do something you enjoy: Life is too short to be on a spin bike if it's not something you enjoy. Start with something you like – cycling outdoors, sea swimming, hillwalking – and along the journey, look at new forms of movement you can include. Always listen to your body: it will tell you what it enjoys, and your mood will tell you too.

Variety is key: Make sure you do different types of exercise throughout your week – ideally a mix of cardio and resistance training. Be open to new movement, especially as you get older. Keeping change a constant in our lives keeps us fresh.

Have a goal: You might want to future-proof your bone health, lose weight or get fitter. Being clear on what you want to achieve will keep you motivated. With my running, I always have a goal in my head: a half marathon, a marathon or to get a quicker time on a 5K. Goals will look different for everyone – an experienced athlete will be aiming for something different from someone getting back into walking. Set goals that will challenge you, and keep stretching them – our bodies love variety and to be pushed to new limits.

Track your movement: A sports watch or fitness tracker can be a handy tool to have. What you want is to be able to monitor your progress, to see the chinks of light coming through and how close you are getting to your goals. The recommendation is to exercise for at least thirty minutes three times per week within your aerobic zone to get the best benefit from aerobic exercise. You can calculate your aerobic zone using your maximum heart rate. This is 220 minus your age (220 is the upper limit of what your cardiovascular system can handle during activity). Your aerobic zone is 70 to 80 per cent of your maximum heart rate – a fitness tracker will help you tell which zone you are in.

Think long term: Ideally, exercise will be a part of your life into the future, so make sure it is sustainable and fits into your lifestyle.

Start slowly and build up: If you have not been taking regular exercise, then start with walking for about twenty minutes, making the last five minutes brisker than the start. You can then begin the brisker walking sooner the next time. You're aiming for thirty minutes of brisk walking altogether. From here you can expand into the many other forms of movement outlined below.

Take time to stretch: Do some stretches for a few minutes in the morning or when taking a break from your desk. After you do any form of exercise, do some gentle stretching.

Make it social: Join a group or start exercising with a friend – this keeps it fun and also means you're more likely to do it for the social aspect. This is a wonderful part of joining an exercise community. You not only get the movement but you get the social interaction too – two of the 6 Ms in one go: movement and mingle.

Recovery is important too: Be mindful of the effects of excessive training on your body. Make sure you take plenty of time to recover and re-energise after exercising, as you don't want to overstretch your muscles and joints or put pressure on your knees.

MOVEMENT FOR THE BODY
Strength training and weights

Including weight-bearing exercises is essential in these years. Every time you do this, you are nourishing your bones and muscles. Sarcopenia, a typical condition of ageing, is the loss of muscle mass, which may occur at a rate of 2 to 3 per cent annually. This can happen from age thirty onwards and is due to being sedentary, but during menopause your declining hormones further accelerate your muscle-mass loss. Strength training should be a vital component of your health through menopause. Adding it to your exercise routine will protect you today – and, more importantly, in the future – from fractures, joint problems and more. Being strong keeps you independent. Work on it – you deserve this and the health it will give, not to mention the confidence.

Remember, too, that strength requires protein, so include this in your diet throughout the day. Without protein, your body won't build muscle, and this building becomes harder in menopause when your body doesn't have the same relationship with protein assimilation as before. Strength training and eating protein will help build and restore muscle.

There are many other benefits of strength training:

- It increases bone strength and builds muscle mass.
- It enables your body to burn calories differently – it uses glucose/energy better, which helps your body combat insulin resistance, heart disease and osteoporosis.
- It improves your posture and heightens your balance and flexibility, which also reduces your risk of falls.
- Feeling strong is fantastic for confidence.
- It boosts your mood, helping you to feel strong mentally as well as physically.
- It can help with the vasomotor symptoms of menopause.

Key for: strength, flexibility, mood and heart health.

Yoga

Yoga is the movement of choice for many women in midlife – its multiple benefits are well documented for mental and physical health. Having a consistent yoga practice gives the most benefits.

You can make it as simple or as challenging as you want. I aim to do about fifteen minutes of yoga three mornings a week and use yoga stretches after running too. I keep it simple: sometimes I use poses I already know; sometimes I refer to a YouTube video or a book – it just depends on what I am in the mood for. There are many different styles of yoga to choose from, from power yoga to restorative yoga, so find out what style suits you best.

These yoga poses are specifically for relaxation and rest: the Child's Pose, the Pigeon, Savasana and, my favourite, the Prayer salute. For more dynamic poses try the Half Sun salute, Warrior lunge, high lunge and dynamic standing twist. Any of these poses are easy to follow and would be a great addition to your daily routine.

Whether it's at home or in your local community centre or gym, yoga is a fabulous movement both for your body and your mind.

Key for: flexibility and mood.

The role of laughter

Laughter yoga – yes, it's a thing and it has moves like 'hot soup', 'cell phones' and 'milkshakes'. Combining laughter, breathing, movement and positivity releases stress and enhances well-being. But you don't have to take a class – laughter is there throughout your day: just look for it. Maybe it's a funny YouTube video; maybe it's over a cuppa with a friend. Find those lighter moments of life that bring joy and fun.

Key for: mood.

Pilates

Pilates is a full-body workout that develops a balance of strength and flexibility within the body. With its focus on breath and mindful execution of the movements, it can help you de-stress as well as build muscular endurance. It's an ideal complementary exercise you can alternate with more cardio-based exercise such as running. Its focus on the inner core, including pelvic floor and diaphragm, can help alleviate symptoms of incontinence and back pain during menopause. Check out both mat and reformer Pilates.

Key for: overall strength and well-being.

Running

Running is one of my personal favourites – I love the headspace it gives me, both during and after a run. The benefits of running are numerous:

- Helps to build strong bones
- Reduces anxiety
- Strengthens muscles
- Improves cardiovascular fitness
- Maintains weight in combination with diet

As with any form of exercise, please start slowly with walking and build up gradually. Use one of the many Couch to 5K apps or websites that provide training programmes for beginners. I highly recommend joining a local running group (I have found so much support and laughter in mine) and – as scary as it might seem – signing up for races and Parkrun events. The community there is second to none.

Key for: mood and heart health.

Walking

Walking in fresh air is the most accessible, easiest and cheapest form of movement, and the physical benefits are many – weight management, heart health, lung capacity and mental health. Whether you walk alone, with a friend or with your dog, you may find your anxiety slowly seeps away.

Key for: mood and heart health.

Forest bathing: shinrin-yoku

The term 'forest bathing', or taking in the forest atmosphere, came from Japan in the 1980s. Whatever its origin, it reinforces what we already know – getting out into nature heals the soul. Recently, a successful study was performed in Donegal called 'The Green Prescription'. It is the first of its kind in Ireland and involves a GP or health professional's referral of patients to free guided community walks. The Green Prescription is based on the idea that physical activity in nature results in positive outcomes for both physical and mental health.

Shinrin-yoku has been scientifically proven to:

- Enhance the immune system and energy levels
- Reduce blood pressure
- Reduce anxiety
- Improve concentration
- Accelerate recovery from sickness
- Aid sleep

Key for: mood.

Dance therapy

Whether alone or with your kids or partner, dancing is a playful, enjoyable way to get movement into your day. And it comes with many emotional, physical and social benefits too.

Dance therapy is a growing field, and whether it's a Zumba class or ballroom dancing, the type of dance is not as important as the feeling it evokes – it should be fun, feel-good and dynamic. Not only does it burn calories, it also relieves stress and stimulates brain cells. Dancing also requires coordination of both your brain and body, which strengthens the neural pathways and improves cognitive function. So drop this book, hit Spotify and get dancing!

Key for: flexibility, mood and heart health.

Breath work

Your breath is always with you, always a ready tool to support you in menopause. Breathing is such a simple exercise and one we often forget the power of. Many women report feeling calmer when they start concentrating more on breathing fully and deeply throughout the day. I believe this is part of the foundation for lessening anxiety and enhancing calm.

This exercise is one to try, commonly referred to as The Rock: sit in a kneeling position with your hands on your knees. Keep your back and arms as straight as possible. Now imagine you are a rock standing totally still in the sea – feel the water swishing around the bottom of you. The water is cool and refreshing. Take in a deep breath of fresh sea air. Each time you breathe in and out, feel your body becoming still and calm.

Key for: calmness, sleep and digestion.

Martial arts

There are many martial arts to choose from – t'ai chi, judo, karate, aikido and taekwondo – and clubs dotted throughout the country.

Key for: flexibility and mood.

Other forms of movement

NEAT, or non-exercise activity thermogenesis, refers to those simple activities we do throughout the day – walking, housework, fidgeting, standing. On a good day, you can burn up to two thousand calories this way, so pick up that pencil and twirl it – fidgeting can be great! A few stretches while you watch Netflix also counts.

Skipping is excellent for balance, agility, coordination and cardiovascular health. Other great cardio exercises are cycling, circuit classes, boxing, tennis, rowing and swimming.

MOVEMENT FOR THE MIND

Mindfulness

Our brains are constantly active and need respite. I see mindfulness as a form of relaxing movement, a movement to nourish your brain.

Mindfulness is well researched for its benefits to our well-being and can be used as a way to train your brain to patiently observe your anxiety. Think of it as if you were a parent observing a toddler's temper tantrum – you can watch the behaviour but need to remain calm and passive until the tantrum is over.

Daily routines can be used as opportunities to practise mindfulness, to focus on the present, on what is happening right now. For mindfulness to become part of your life, it must work for you. It must be something you benefit from and not something you dread. In that respect, start small and let it find ways into your life. When sitting in traffic, just *be* for a few moments, right where you are, not on the way to somewhere or the way from somewhere, not late, not early. Just there, in that moment.

When we stop and sit in 'the now', we can slow down what we are experiencing and take time to savour and enjoy what life has to offer. Being mindful lets our minds be present and become clearer. The realisation that this very moment is all there is – everything else is merely a thought, projected into the future or excavated from the past – is the start of letting go of worry. Stress fades away and our minds become calmer. It's all about taking life in smaller bites, not hour by hour but minute by minute. Just focus on the next sixty seconds.

Begin with simple ways to be present:

- Making tea – slow down and pay attention to the movement of your hands, the smell of the tea, the steam from the kettle, the sound of the water pouring and, finally, the taste of the tea.
- Washing your hands – pay attention to the water, the smell of the

soap, the slipperiness of the lather and the movement and sensation of your fingers and palms. Pay attention to only these things for a few moments – this is a sort of meditation.

- Eating – notice the textures, the colours and the aroma of your food as well as the taste; slow down the action of eating and focus on the sensation of the food on your palate.
- Do a digital detox for an hour during the day.

Meditation

Like many meditation novices, I took a long time to develop the habit and to see the benefits. But when I persevered, I discovered that the same principle applied to meditation as to movement for the physical body: repetition and practice increase strength. You don't need to be sitting cross-legged like the famous yogis; you can meditate anywhere that works for you. The benefits of meditation are widely celebrated, and once you find what works for you it is a great addition to your daily habits. I try to do mine first thing in the morning, and it is an excellent way to start the day, but there are times that doesn't happen and then I squeeze it in where I can. And, yes, there are days I don't manage it at all, but I always go back to it.

When I started meditation I really struggled. Most people do. Emptying your head of thoughts is a tough challenge for the busy minds we have developed. From what to cook for dinner, to a conversation at work, to an itchy nose – all kinds of random thoughts infiltrated my first attempts. Think of your meditation time as a way of destressing – watching these thoughts pass by is unloading some of that stress and anxiety.

Start small – five minutes is enough per day to get you started. You can use apps (Insight, Calm and Headspace are all great), YouTube channels or other guided meditations if you like – find what works for you. I have done some of my most amazing meditating sitting on a bench or a rock up in the mountains. Make it fit into your life and create a space for it – you will never regret it. Every time you meditate, you are changing pathways in your brain; you are reshaping and protecting yourself for the future.

Sleep and movement

In Chapter 4 we talked about sleep being the bedrock of thriving through menopause. If you exercise with little to no sleep, your body will be more resistant. If you exercise from a depleted state, it will do you no favours – it will, in fact, put more stress on your body and encourage more cortisol production, which we're trying to reduce. Lack of sleep and restless nights impact not only cortisol but also melatonin and insulin (your blood sugar hormone). If cortisol is high, the overnight fat-burning activity in your body is impacted. It also means you won't recover as well from any exercise you have been doing, and deep tiredness can set in.

It's essential to get the balance right – get sleep sorted first and then start to work on movement. A stressed body is not good for you: it encourages inflammation and exhaustion. Sleep first, movement second.

* * *

Look for every opportunity in your day to move – it may be taking the stairs instead of the lift, walking while you take a phone call or parking further away from work or the shops so you can get a walk in. If you're ever in doubt, just remember all the benefits movement brings to your life – improved mood, weight management, lower insulin, heart health and fun!

And remember, these movements are to improve your life, not to add any additional form of stress. Be kind to yourself, make small changes and do what works best for you.

19

Menu – the importance of good food

I adore food. I love eating it, cooking it, looking at it, you name it. I have a deep respect for food, too, and for those who grow and produce what we all enjoy every day.

What you eat determines how well your body fares. Eat good food and your body will shine, sparkle and thank you. What we put into our bodies directly affects our moods and emotions. You can follow a good exercise routine, practise mindfulness and use medication, but the full benefits will be lost if nutrition is not part of your plan. A properly balanced diet will enhance your energy levels, may provide relief from many symptoms of your menopause and is also part of future-proofing your body.

'We are what we eat.' It's as simple as that. A diet with high levels of sugar and processed foods will cause mood swings, energy spikes and crashes, weight gain and sluggishness. Anxiety, stress, tension and tiredness can all be alleviated by a good, balanced diet. When we look at food, we also need to consider gut health, immunity and the health of the liver and, as discussed in Chapter 10, the role of insulin.

Food is very personal and if you are experiencing ongoing issues related to food this is an excellent time in your life to work with a dietitian or nutritional therapist to ensure you are including the key foods in your daily diet.

IT ALL STARTS IN THE GUT

I like to think of the gut as a garden – when it is flourishing, so is your mind. Ample research has been done on the gut–brain connection, and it is now accepted that the two are directly linked, with the gut sometimes being referred to as 'the second brain'. We know the gut is responsible for producing a large amount of the body's neurotransmitters, those vital messengers (chemicals) that send information from the brain to the body and vice versa via the vagus nerve, which I think is underrated when it comes to stress and anxiety – about 80 to 95 per cent of serotonin is produced in the gut. The stomach is also our first line of defence against illness, providing a barrier to ward off viruses and bacteria.

We all know long-term ongoing exposure to stress is a contributing factor to many illnesses. In today's world, we have to buffer ourselves against many types of stress that weren't in existence ten or twenty years ago.

To fully understand how chronic stress impacts our bodies, we need to look at the gastrointestinal tract (gut). When we talk about the gut, we talk about the microbiome. This is its own mini ecosystem with a collection of microorganisms, not just a place for digesting food and absorbing nutrients. So much more happens here.

A staggering 80 per cent of our immune system is located in the gut. When you have a stomach upset, when you're not feeling well, when you're anxious, experiencing on–off constipation, you must look to your gut. Your gut has over a hundred trillion bacteria that are vital to maintaining a healthy body. They are the soldiers defending against the bad bacteria that make your body ill.

Finally, in understanding the gut, a key part is permeability. Basically, what separates everything in the gut from going into our bloodstream is one layer of cells. This layer lining the gut needs to be very strong to block bad bacteria from entering the bloodstream while still allowing nutrients to pass through into the blood: that's a big job. When this lining breaks down, it's called leaky gut/increased gut permeability and it can wreak havoc on our bodies.

Under stress, the brain triggers the 'sympathetic response' to protect itself, and this is when the gut lining becomes compromised. This fight-or-flight response robs blood from the gut and moves it to the limbs, so that you can run from the perceived danger. Today's world has a huge amount of ongoing stress and anxiety that triggers the sympathetic response and contributes to gut permeability.

It's imperative to look after your gut health. And that requires feeding and nourishing the 'garden' so that everything flourishes. This is where good bacteria (probiotics and prebiotics) come into play.

Probiotics

Probiotics are important and not only for digestion and good gut health – they reach much further across our entire bodies. The two key players, *Lactobacillus* and bifidobacteria, have been shown to have antiviral properties and may help reduce the length of a viral respiratory infection. Probiotics produce antibodies, which attach to foreign or unknown bacteria or viruses to encourage your white blood cells to attack them. White blood cells are key in helping the body fight against viruses and bacteria. I often meet women who are experiencing low white blood count during the menopause years – this is something to watch for in your regular blood tests.

Probiotics are found in highest quantities in fermented foods (for example, yogurt, milk kefir, kombucha, kimchi and sauerkraut).

Prebiotics

Prebiotics are like fertilisers for probiotics, the essential ingredients to make your garden bloom. The more prebiotics in your gut, the healthier your probiotics, gut and immune system will be. Good sources of prebiotics include lentils, beans, garlic, leeks, bananas, broccoli, beetroot, parsnips, onions, artichokes and oats. Prebiotics naturally exist in many foods we consume on a daily basis, and as fibre is a source of prebiotics, foods high in fibre are usually high in prebiotics.

YOUR RACING CAR

When looking at what we eat each day, it is helpful to understand the importance of the neurotransmitters in our bodies and their interaction with the key glands – adrenal and pituitary. Think of your body as a racing car and your food as the fuel to recharge: without the right fuel, your body cannot provide optimum healthy performance. The fuel creates energy, which links and interacts with all parts of your body, with the most important parts being the brain and the gut. The brain will send messages to different parts of the body when required, using neurotransmitters. How we fuel (feed) our bodies is key to our physical and mental health.

YOUR LIVER

In traditional Chinese medicine, 'free and easy wanderer' refers to someone who is flowing in the 'stream of life' and not going against the current. In perimenopause, and at other times, we can often feel we are going upstream against a strong current, which leads to intense moods that change like the wind. Frustration, irritability, anger, depression and anxiety – all of these emotions and feelings show what is going on in our lives, but they may also point to the liver being out of balance. I see this a lot with women I talk to – we often forget our livers and the major role they perform in our bodies.

The liver and kidneys work closely together when we look at the energy in our bodies, and this relationship is at its peak in perimenopause. An imbalance in one affects the other. If the liver is not getting the nourishment it needs, this can affect your periods, digestion, immunity, libido, sleep and, more importantly, your moods and your mind.

The job of the liver

The liver is a powerhouse – it is a constant hub of activity and performs hundreds of jobs to ensure you are healthy. It helps to store fuel for when you need more energy (remember, it's a back-up reserve for insulin) and helps to balance blood glucose levels. It is like a filtration system that helps clean your blood and keep it toxin free. It also helps with blood clotting and stores certain vitamins. The work it undertakes around the clock to synthesise your hormones is crucial in perimenopause. If your liver is unhappy, it will reflect in tiredness, itchy skin, aching joints, fuzzy head, hot flushes and constipation, to name just a few.

The liver is a storehouse for some key vitamins – mainly vitamin A (eyesight, bones, teeth, skin and hair); vitamin D (bones and especially for mood); vitamin K (blood clotting – vital in perimenopause if you're suffering from heavy periods or flooding); vitamin B12 (the best support for your nervous system – also for energy levels, memory and concentration); and iron (immunity and tiredness).

Last but not least, the liver is important for hormones. When our hormones have completed their role in the body, they are sent to the liver. Your liver needs to be functioning optimally to ensure that detoxification happens. Otherwise, you end up with more hormones in your body than should be there. One important role of the liver is the excretion and recycling of hormones.

What else can I do to help my liver?
After eating nourishing, supportive foods – plenty of vegetables and fresh fruit – a great way to cleanse your liver is with the herb milk thistle. Its antioxidant and anti-inflammatory properties make it a great friend of the liver. It is worth taking this for a month at a time to detox and nourish your liver – make sure to take it away from food to get the optimum benefits.

BE REGULAR – THE IMPORTANCE OF A DAILY POO
A vital step in supporting your body through menopause is ensuring a daily bowel movement that is easy and causes no straining or discomfort, with the feeling of the bowel being totally empty. This helps your immunity, as it ensures toxins are released from your body and your energy is kept flowing as it should. The very act of eating creates a wave-like effect that moves waste through our

bodies down to our bowels. It has long been ingrained to ignore these messages, so our digestive system becomes sluggish. If you think of a baby or young child, they will generally have a bowel movement after each meal. This changes as we get older – we hold on and control this process more. However, please ensure you go to the toilet when you need to and don't put it off: this is not good for your body and can in time lead to constipation.

Constipation is when you are not having daily bowel movements and may result in hard, dry stools which are difficult to pass. Many women will experience constipation during these years and some may have IBS-like symptoms as well. These include constipation, diarrhoea, bloating, stomach cramps and wind. IBS is very common and can be exacerbated by the additional stress that menopause might bring. Changes in oestrogen levels can impact how your gut operates and increased cortisol production plays a role here too.

The speed at which fuel, your food, travels through your body is important, too. That time from the starting line to the finish – from food going into your mouth to exiting in the toilet – the faster, the better. Some foods have quicker times, others slower. Fibre is your best friend here, as it is quickest to the finish line. Other foods, like meat, are slower.

Water is essential in ensuring good bowel health. Regular drinks of water throughout the day will also keep your body hydrated. Ensure a plentiful diet of wholegrains, fruit and vegetables to get the fibre you need.

If you are experiencing ongoing symptoms of IBS and changes in your diet are not helping, please seek advice from your doctor and/or a dietitian.

HOW WE EAT

Eating on the go, breakfast at the counter – we don't sit as much as we used to. Having a healthy diet is only one step when it comes to feeding your body good sources of fuel. How and when you eat it is just as important.

Do you really feel hungry?

It's OK to be hungry – it's actually not a bad thing to feel that rumbling in your tummy. When it reaches a peak, don't worry, because your fabulous brain will send a clear message to you to get some food (the hunger hormone ghrelin). You know when you're driving your car and it beeps to tell you to refuel or recharge? Your brain does the exact same for your body. This is real, raw hunger.

This can be helpful when you're trying to figure out whether you are actually hungry or just bored. This is very common. So the starting point is understanding your body and the message it is sending you. You also don't need to clear your plate at every meal. As adults, we are more aware of what we are eating, and you can take control and tell yourself that it's OK to leave food on your plate if you feel full.

Eating mindfully

Taking time over food is so important. Are you a chewer or do you just gulp your food down? Chewing is good for us: it breaks down the food and makes our digestive system's job much easier. It also helps to make you feel full faster. Take the time to enjoy and chew each mouthful. Ideally, we should chew each mouthful twenty times before swallowing.

How often have you eaten food, only seconds after to not even remember how it tasted? How often do you forget what you ate because it was consumed so fast? Be conscious of how your food tastes and how it feels in your mouth. We are sensory beings and there is nothing more sensory than enjoying good food.

Heartburn, which is acid reflux, can also happen in these years. Here, the acid that should be in your stomach comes up into the windpipe, causing a burning sensation. Changes to food and how you eat can help with this symptom.

WHEN TO EAT

My favourite meal of the day is breakfast – I am always starving when I wake up. But many women tell me that they skip this essential start to the day. I would encourage you to revisit this if it's the case for you. Breakfast generally comes after several hours of sleep, where the body has had an opportunity to fast and clean itself up and is ready with fresh energy. Ensure good protein intake in your first meal of the day, as this is an excellent start for your overall muscle health.

When it comes to evening time, the longer you can let your body fast overnight the better – ideally a minimum of twelve hours. If you are an evening snacker, try to have healthy snacks rather than crisps and chocolate. Some nuts and natural yogurt can be a lovely evening treat.

But, remember, it's all about listening to your body, as we are all different when it comes to hunger levels – eat when *you* feel hungry.

> Food saved me. I was not a good eater until I got the loud wake-up call of menopause. Brain fog, being constantly hot, crippling anxiety and low moods. Jesus, I couldn't drive on the M50 for months with my anxiety. And my weight was just getting heavier. I joined a weight-loss group, but couldn't sustain it. I started to watch and track what I ate every day and, in a funny way, I can thank my menopause for my new appreciation of food. Now I focus daily on food, and two years later I can tell you with a big smile I am pretty much symptom free. I put it down to food and daily exercise.
>
> – Claire

WHAT TO EAT

The old adage 'you are what you eat' is never more true than in menopause. Several key aspects are important to be particularly mindful of in these years.

Protein

Oestrogen changes in menopause have a link to decreased muscle and bone strength. Protein has an important role to play in your muscle and bone health. Being composed of amino acids, it is responsible for the production of hormones, enzymes and antibodies. Amino acids are a key part of the daily upkeep of your body – your digestive health, immunity and brain health. As muscle loss occurs with ageing and menopause, it is important to have a good supply of protein in your diet to boost this. Protein has the added advantage of making you feel fuller. The key is not to go all-in here but to have a steady moderate intake.

Ideally, you are aiming for a minimum of 0.8g per kg of your weight per day if you are moderately active; if you are doing intense training, you will need more: 1.2–2g per kg of body weight.

But let's be practical – it's hard to measure this every day, so aim for the size of your palm as a good portion. If it's yogurt or beans, then a small cupful will be about the same. Having protein at each meal is ideal, as you are spreading its effect throughout the day.

High protein foods are eggs, meat, fish, beans, nuts, seeds (hemp seeds are mighty), grains, tofu, soy and dairy products. If you are obtaining your protein from plant sources, you will need a greater volume to get the same amount of grams of protein. It's important to include grains and beans to ensure you get the full variety of amino acids in your diet. Beans are a super protein food. They are full of fibre, help you feel full for longer and help maintain blood sugar levels. Dan Brutter's research on the Blue Zones – those regions of the world where people live longer – tells us that some of the longest-living people in the world eat a cup of beans a day. That's evidence enough for me! Remember, though, that beans equal wind, so add them to your diet slowly. Soaking them and long cooking help too.

As with all food sources, the trick is to get variety in your daily intake, which will ensure you are consuming the key amino acids.

Protein powders can also have a role to play, but be mindful of the ingredients included. Ideally, you are looking for the main protein source to come from whey, soy, pea or brown rice.

The complexity of carbohydrates

We tend to run a mile when we see or hear about carbs. But your body needs carbohydrates: we need the glucose that comes from these foods. Glucose is our bodies' main energy source.

There are two main groups: simple and complex carbohydrates. How your food is made structurally determines whether it is simple or complex. Complex carbs – starches and fibre – are less likely to cause spikes in your blood sugar levels, and contain vitamins, minerals and the all fibre we need. Simple carbs are absorbed quickly into the bloodstream, resulting in a quick boost of energy (not always a bad thing). But not all simple carbs contain beneficial vitamins and minerals, as discussed below, and can cause weight gain (insulin spikes) and increase your risk of diabetes, heart disease and high cholesterol.

What are starches?

Many starches are complex carbohydrates, but not all. As with all complex carbohydrates, it takes longer for your body to break them down. That means they are good for your blood sugar levels, keeping them stable, providing energy over a sustained period of time, and also making you feel fuller for longer.

Sources: Beans, legumes, fruits like apples, berries, whole grains, brown rice, oatmeal and vegetables like corn, peas and potatoes.

What are sugars?

Sugars are simple carbohydrates, so your body will break down these foods faster. This makes blood sugar levels rise – and then drop – very quickly. That's the quick hit you get from sugary foods, followed soon by an energy drain.

Labelling is important here, as foods often contain hidden sugars, so take the time to read the ingredients closely. There are two forms of sugars to be conscious of: those that occur naturally in foods, such as in milk and fresh fruit; and added sugars, which are ingredients in most processed foods and drinks.

Your body doesn't know the difference between naturally occurring and processed sugars. It processes them the same way. The difference to be aware of is that the naturally occurring sugars also have vitamins and minerals and, in some cases, fibre.

You may see sugar listed in many ways, with sugar, cane syrup, corn syrup, dextrose, fructose, sucrose, maple syrup, honey, molasses or agave nectar being some key ones.

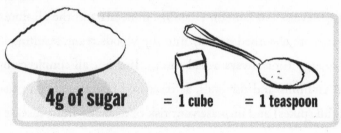

A higher position on the ingredients list on a food label indicates that more of an ingredient is contained within the product. Also watch out for 'carbohydrates of which sugar': this shows how much sugar per 100g the product contains. Anything over 15g is high, and less than 5g is low. Sugar is one of the biggest nutrient robbers, so I would encourage you to monitor and limit your sugar intake as much as possible.

Please note that other forms of simple carb are fruits, milk and milk products.

What is fibre?

Fibre is another complex carbohydrate. Your body cannot break down fibre (it's the non-digestible component of plants) so most of it just passes through, but it does great work on the way. It is essential for digestive and bowel health, stimulating and helping digestion as it moves through your body. It also helps to maintain blood sugar levels, give a feeling of fullness and lower cholesterol. Most people have far less fibre in their diet than they should – ideally, consuming 25–30g per day is the target. You also will come across soluble and non-soluble fibre – fibre that dissolves in water (such as in psyllium husks and oats) and fibre that doesn't (such as in wholemeal flour, almonds and walnuts). Your body needs both and, again, variety is key here. Fibre also has a positive impact on weight management, helping you feel fuller for longer and supporting positive insulin production.

Sources: Beans, lentils, fruits, nuts and seeds, whole grains and vegetables.

Hydration

We delved into this in Chapter 8, as it has such a big impact on brain fog. I would encourage you to make hydration your starting point. Dehydration will only add to your symptoms. So drink extra water – aim for a minimum of six to eight glasses across your day. You can *eat* your water – include foods that are high in water content, like watermelon and cucumbers.

A cup of herbal tea also counts – there are many to choose from: turmeric, hot water and lemon, green tea (this can contain caffeine, so maybe avoid at night-time), sage (great for hot flushes) and valerian (particularly at night-time). I am a great fan of tulsi tea also.

It's important to absorb the water you drink, rather than just flush out your system. To enhance hydration, add the following to your diet: coconut water, watermelon, celery, kefir, yogurt, cucumber, kiwi, bell pepper, citrus fruits, carrot and pineapple.

Phytoestrogens

These are plant-derived compounds found in several foods and are split into four groups: isoflavones, flavonoids, stilbenes and lignans. As the name suggests, they mimic the action of oestrogen in the body but on a very different level to synthetic HRT, binding to oestrogen receptors in the body. They can be very beneficial for the heart and bones.

Current research shows soy isoflavones may have a positive impact on hot flushes. How effective soy is in your body is also linked to your gut bacteria, namely the production of equol, which has been linked with fewer symptoms of menopause. The important thing is to look at the right food source. Fermented soy products are the best. As soy is a complete protein, regular intake is linked with improved heart health.

The best sources of phytoestrogens to use on a daily basis are flaxseeds, chickpeas, soy, tofu, edamame beans, alfalfa and peanuts. If your diet contains fruits, vegetables, legumes and some grains, then you are already getting phytoestrogens. A plant-based diet is very rich in natural phytoestrogens in healthy amounts, especially from soy.

Potential benefits of phytoestrogens may include:

- Reducing menopausal hot flushes
- Preventing bone loss and protecting against osteoporosis
- Stabilising blood sugar levels
- Regulating the menstrual cycle
- Possible improving of cognitive function

The average Asian diet contains 40–80mg of phytoestrogens per day, while in the US and Europe, it's 3mg per day or less. This may be why Asian women, and Japanese women in particular, do not experience the variety of symptoms that women in the West do. You can also increase your intake of phytoestrogens through supplements containing red clover. These can be beneficial for many of the typical symptoms of menopause.

Herbs and spices

Introduce these every way you can in these years. Cinnamon is very easy to add to your food and may help balance blood sugar levels. Saffron has been linked to supporting balanced mood. Sage is good for reducing hot flushes. Rosemary may help with cognition. Ginger, pepper and turmeric are helpful additions for energy. A world of discovery – and flavour – awaits with herbs and spices!

Supporting progesterone through diet

No food products contain progesterone. However, certain foods may support the body's production of progesterone. More clinical research is required in this area.

NUTRIENT ROBBERS – FOODS TO LIMIT

Processed foods

Raw, untouched foods contain the most nutrients and this is why, for most vegetables, it is best to just steam them ever so slightly. Processed foods do not provide the same nutrients as freshly cooked foods. They generally need additives and preservatives to keep them fresh, and they tend to be low in fibre and protein. Ideally, food is grown to be eaten from the field to the plate. As with everything, moderation is key.

Caffeine

Our tolerance to caffeine is individual, with some of us more sensitive to it than others. And caffeine does have benefits, just in moderation. We know that drinking caffeine can be beneficial to heart health when you limit it to three cups per day. (See also Chapter 4.)

Sugar

This is by far one of the biggest culprits, as discussed above.

Alcohol

I can't talk about alcohol without again mentioning the importance of the liver. I see the liver as the body's ultimate protector from illness and disease. It works constantly. And alcohol is not your or your liver's friend in menopause. To this day I still love and appreciate a good red wine. However, as I have gotten older I have become more sensitive to alcohol – this is very common and happens to many people (see Chapter 3 for more on histamine intolerance).

The liver is our storehouse of antioxidants – vitamin C and the B vitamins. Magnesium and iron are also stored here, and these are crucial at every stage in life. Alcohol depletes these stores and therefore depletes your body's store of these essential vitamins and minerals. Men process alcohol through their bodies much faster than women – our bodies work it through at a slower rate, and so the side effects last longer.

Alcohol is a depressant – there's no way around this. Drinking alcohol puts added stress on your adrenal glands, it increases the stress hormone cortisol and, after an initial rush, leaves you feeling low and tired. It disrupts your blood sugar levels, which, as we have seen, are essential to keep stable in menopause. Often alcohol is used as a coping mechanism, and while it may temporarily dampen symptoms, it will exacerbate them in the long term.

Alcohol also lowers your body's ability to absorb calcium – another essential nutrient for our body and bones – and causes increased blood pressure.

Sometimes women tell me a glass of wine helps them sleep better at night. It might put you to sleep quicker, but you may not get the good night's sleep that you would otherwise. You may find you wake up at some point in the night and then are unable to return to sleep, or when it's time to get up you feel exhausted and drained.

Alcohol is also very dehydrating, and if you are already getting night sweats or hot flushes, then drinking alcohol regularly is going to compound the problem. It also heightens anxiety. If you are experiencing any levels of anxiety, I would strongly encourage you to minimise alcohol consumption.

The recommendation for women is to consume fewer than eleven standard drinks spread out over the week, with two alcohol-free days at minimum. A standard drink contains 10g of pure alcohol.

I know it is unrealistic in many cases to say stop alcohol consumption altogether, but where the symptoms are severe, you do need to consider how quickly you want to feel better and get back to enjoying life.

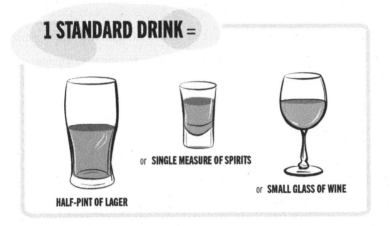

1 STANDARD DRINK =

HALF-PINT OF LAGER

or SINGLE MEASURE OF SPIRITS

or SMALL GLASS OF WINE

Smoking

If you are a smoker, I would love you to consider a quitting programme to help you to stop. There is no benefit to smoking, only downsides – earlier menopause, lung cancer, heart issues and cost, to name but a few.

IS A PLANT-BASED DIET ESSENTIAL IN MENOPAUSE?

There is good evidence to support that a plant-based diet can be beneficial for many aspects of menopause, but it is not for everyone. Recent studies also support reducing red meat consumption in these years. I still eat red meat, although a lot less than I used to.

An animal-based diet contains animal fat and animal hormones (more in some countries than others) and is slower for the body to digest. A plant-based diet, being higher in fibre, moves more quickly through the body, which is a good thing. This topic can be further complicated by looking at protein: animal and plant protein sources will offer different amino acids. A variety of these is important and this can be more easily achieved through an animal-based diet (remember how important protein is for our muscle health).

COST OF FOOD

Our shopping will vary greatly for each of us, according to what we can afford, and when it comes to organic produce, it's good to know the 'dirty dozen' – those fruits and vegetables that can be higher in pesticides. A great tip here is to clean non-organic produce in white vinegar and water – place the vegetables in a bowl containing four parts water to one part vinegar and soak for 20 minutes. You can then rinse them and let them dry off.

* * *

What you eat is personal, it will be based on many factors – including what is affordable and manageable for you – and rarely be specific to menopause. The most important thing is to know your downfalls and make small changes to your daily habits. Small changes will last. For me, it's the 80:20 rule. It's OK to have lapses – just try to make nutrition choices that you can support 80 per cent of the time. We can't spend our lives being good every minute, so if you can adopt this rule, it's a great start.

We are all unique in this journey, and we will all experience different symptoms and challenges along the way. Listen to your body and what it is telling you, and make your choices based on these internal signals. Our bodies send us symptoms to tell us what needs attention and to help us on the journey.

20

Mingle – connection with others

Would you ride a rollercoaster all by yourself? I wouldn't, because the thrill is in the squeals you get from riding it with someone else. Menopause is one of those experiences that is better with a group of companions, a support network.

Today, life is very busy. Between travel, work, technology and just day-to-day living, it can be hard to carve out time for each other. Menopause can be isolating, and it's a time when you'll need help from many people in your life.

The loneliness and isolation can be exacerbated by social anxiety, in which you have a persistent fear of social settings and being around other people. These sensations are more severe and overwhelming than shyness. It might be where a specific circumstance, such as going to the cinema or eating in a restaurant, provokes anxiety, or it can be more general, where anxiety arises as a result of any situation with a social component.

Women in their forties and in perimenopause are more likely to experience social anxiety disorder than men. This is explained or aggravated in part by the social issues of perimenopause, such as heavy periods and potentially humiliating flooding episodes, intense hot flushes and the sweating that accompanies them. Brain fog can actually cause women to forget names and dates, which can be distressing in social circumstances or at work. All of these factors, together with the changes in body shape associated with the forties and fifties, can lead to low self-esteem and self-confidence, which may lead to social anxiety.

Also, even though you may be in a relationship, if that relationship is not fulfilling or meaningful this can also trigger a sense of loneliness and isolation. In many cases, feeling lonely within a relationship can bring with it a host of painful and upsetting feelings. And chances are menopause might shine a light on this too. Loneliness can be exacerbated when a person feels misunderstood or feels different from others, which can often be the case in menopause.

The 2019 Irish TILDA study found that almost one-third of adults over fifty in Ireland experienced emotional loneliness some of the time and 7 per cent often felt lonely. Poor health and chronic conditions were associated with higher levels of loneliness. The study also found that the link between loneliness and depression was much stronger than the association between social isolation and depression.

There are also health aspects of feeling lonely, with it being closely correlated to cognitive decline and bringing an increased risk of heart issues and obesity, and with the World Health Organisation listing 'social support networks' as a key determinant of overall health.

Sadly, loneliness can be felt acutely in menopause. This is the time to reach out and get your A-team in place – your tribe.

I was totally unprepared, ill-informed and never heard of the term perimenopause when I was ambushed by unpleasant symptoms three months to my fiftieth birthday. From then on, I started out on this journey of educating and researching everything to do with the topic. Unfortunately, menopause has been a setback and total inconvenience to my life. Despite more conversation and the topic becoming more mainstream, many of us are suffering in silence as the taboo remains quite strong among our generation. For example, I myself have five younger sisters between the ages of forty-six and fifty-four and the taboo is alive and kicking, which I find upsetting, to be honest. One of the hardest aspects of menopause is the loneliness and isolation of it all! It's so unfair and awful how we become more withdrawn and anti-social.

– Brigid

FINDING YOUR TRIBE

It takes a village to raise a child, so the saying goes. I also believe it takes a community to support a woman going through menopause.

The Okinawans, who live in one of the world's most renowned Blue Zone countries, have a concept known as Moai. This refers to a small group of friends that form a tribe and watch out for one another throughout their lives. They understand the importance of connection and the influence it has on their health and life.

Sit down and think about who is in your tribe, who you can confide in. Talking about your experience and your feelings will give you a sense of perspective and lighten the load. And talking with someone you like and trust, and offering them support too, can deepen your connection. Surround yourself with positive people, those with the capacity to listen and to support, and avoid those who sap your energy or bring you down in any way.

FAMILY

Partners, children and extended family members will go through menopause with you. They just might not know what is happening. This is why it can be of great benefit to you and those close to you to share what you are experiencing. Without talking, they will be left in the dark and not understand what is going on. I would also encourage you to chat to other family members about it – I often hear from women who say their female relatives never discussed it, and they are now trying to open up the subject. Also, if you have children, they may have little to no knowledge of menopause (until such time as we have it added to the school curriculum), and understanding menopause will enable them to understand compassionately what you are experiencing and what they may experience one day. Menopause doesn't just impact the person going through it: it affects all those their life touches on.

How to start the conversation with your partner

What you don't want to do is wait for all your frustration, rage and upset to pour out in a flood of anger and words you will regret. Ideally, you want to approach it so your partner understands what you are feeling. Most partners feel adrift and isolated in these years, not understanding why their partners have changed so much. And your partner may see the change before you do. Menopause is a time when a woman may become quiet, may reassess and look inward more than before. This is part of the transformative process that it brings. And this is when you want your partner on your side.

Writing a letter, even an email if that's more your thing, can be a good place to start if you are anxious about a face-to-face conversation – or pass them this book and ask them to read Chapter 23. This can lay the groundwork for the chat about what you are experiencing. Many partners are relieved when they hear what's going on, as often they feel they must have done something wrong.

FRIENDS

My favourite day of the week is Friday, which starts with an early morning run and then the best bit: a long coffee with my running pals. It's a complete unfiltered kick-back, and it's me without any role. I'm not a mum, not a menopause advocate, I'm just me. When you spend time like this with people, all aspects of your life are chatted about, you go through highs and lows together, and there is always laughter. Friends who know you well, who you can be yourself with, are integral now.

We all have friends we know we can fall back on and rely on, from exercise groups to college, school and work friends. Those are the people who support you, who you have the best laughs with and you know you can always trust.

As we grow older, clarity emerges, and you may find yourself having to say goodbye to connections that no longer serve you as well as they once did. Relationships that are both supportive and nurturing are exactly what you require right now, not negativity.

Online groups are a wonderful resource too – particularly for those who find it difficult, for whatever reasons, to do things outside the home – and there are plenty to pick from. Just use your common sense and make sure it's a supportive environment free of fear-based, one-sided viewpoints. You want a welcoming environment with a variety of viewpoints.

WORKPLACE SUPPORT

Many workplaces are starting forums and monthly get-togethers for co-workers to discuss their menopause in a confidential setting. This is fantastic to see, and if you're comfortable doing so, it could be another terrific opportunity to meet new people and share your experiences. Don't forget the support your workplace EAP can offer too.

PSYCHOLOGICAL AND MEDICAL SUPPORTS

As discussed earlier and throughout the book, these will be your GP, your women's health physiotherapist and, if you think it would help, a therapist.

SIMPLE STEPS TO STAY CONNECTED

Expand your connections: step outside your current comfort zone – new friendships can be developed and this will benefit you in many ways.

Plan it: find the time each week to stay connected with those close to you.

Meet in person: nothing beats sitting or walking with a friend in person. If you can, leave the phone in your bag and be totally present. Alternatively, a video chat will also provide that much-needed eye contact and face time if going out is not an option.

Phone a friend just to say hello: instead of a text, pick up the phone and reach out – not because you need something or something is going on, but simply because you want to.

Become a regular: join a group or a club, and make it a habit to attend – you will form new friendships and this will be nourishing for you on many levels. Make it local and become part of the community.

Envision a positive experience: it may feel scary initially, especially if you're trying new groups, but be curious about who you might meet and what you might learn, and think of the best possible outcome.

* * *

Staying socially connected plays an important role in your overall health. Not only does it help to keep the neurotransmitters in your brain firing on all cylinders but it also keeps you happier and healthier. Dr Rangan Chatterjee suggests we aim for one new friendship each year, and I think this is a wonderful way to approach life at any stage, bringing a newness and fresh perspective to your experience.

21

Meaning – finding your joy

Viktor Frankl, a holocaust survivor, believed that no matter what is going on in your life, you have an opportunity to find meaning. If you have meaning, he stated, you will live longer: having purpose is more important than having wealth and education. Menopause is a period of reassessment, and an integral part of this is nourishing those aspects of your life that bring you joy and contentment.

But how does this work when you're running on empty, when sleep is evasive and you're a whirlwind of emotions? Well, there is always a chink, a spark of meaning that may be small and hidden, and bringing together all you have learned in relation to your menopause will start to allow the light to stream in. You are now steering your own ship.

Psychologist Murray Stein writes that midlife brings attention to needs or desires that have been repressed, and women need to integrate the pieces of themselves that have been missing to make them whole – a return to your true self. During midlife, people gain a new understanding of their limits and develop a new sense of meaning. Many women in midlife start to ask questions about meaning, purpose and fulfilment – you may start to ponder where you are in your life.

IKIGAI – YOUR PASSION OR PURPOSE IN LIFE

The Blue Zones study of countries that have the longest life spans has highlighted essential aspects of life that promote healthy living and longevity. Chief among them is 'ikigai', a Japanese term for your passion, your purpose in life.

Ikigai has many dimensions, but the source is knowing or finding your passion, an ingredient in your life that completes you in a healthy way. Cultivating your passions will support and nurture your mental and physical self. It could be learning a musical instrument, your job, cooking, exercising (within moderation) or learning a new language – the sky's the limit.

Your menopause wants you to find and enjoy activities that make you smile – that will make you happy and give zest to your life. I have met many women who have changed direction in their menopause years, either through a career change, taking up a new hobby, starting a new form of exercise or finding a new aspect to their lives.

And this new addition or cultivation of a current activity you love will be one you become easily immersed in – time fades, and you are lost in the moment, in a state of flow.

Five years ago I was coerced into joining a local art class. I had never drawn or painted before, but I was always interested in art and visiting exhibitions and galleries. I was very apprehensive at first but, having a wonderful teacher who inspired and encouraged me, I was soon hooked. For the past two years I've been attending a course every Wednesday. It's the highlight of my week – I absolutely love it. I've made great new friends and have gained confidence in not being afraid to try new things. I also volunteer in our local gallery. I paint every spare second and couldn't care less about housework. If you'd told me twenty years ago this is what I'd be doing, there's no way I'd have believed you!

– Paula

HOW TO UNLOCK YOUR MEANING

What do you really enjoy doing? Where do you lose time and the hours fly by? What are you passionate about?

This is individual and personal to each of us, just like our entire menopause journey. It may already be there and you are enjoying it – now, maybe you can think about expanding on it further. Or maybe you're not sure what it is – if that's the case, it's easy to uncover. It just takes some time and patience.

The first step is to think about what you enjoy. This can be when you're sitting in the car or having a cup of tea – just whenever you have some headspace to sit with yourself. A lovely way is to dedicate fifteen minutes each week to sitting down, putting pen to paper and thrashing out your thoughts. You will be amazed what comes over a few weeks. Often your own life's experience will lead you on this path. My experience of perimenopause is how I started doing the work I do, my passion rooted in my own personal journey.

It does not have to be a job change, though – it can be any aspect of your life. Just be open to what comes up as you start to think more about this.

As Walter Breuning, who lived to 114 years, said, 'If you keep your mind and body busy, you'll be around a long time.'

Starting a lifestyle blog at fifty-eight was a huge challenge. But I wanted to share my experiences, open up the conversation around ageing, encourage women to live life to the full. Don't be afraid to go outside your comfort zone; embrace new experiences and find joy in the little things.

– Hilda Smith

22

Minding you – crucial care

How often do you put others first and put yourself last, prioritising the needs of friends and family over your own? Menopause wants you to take care of yourself – it requires it. This isn't about self-care: it's about crucial care, about carving out some time for yourself. There is no self-centeredness here. If you don't take care of yourself now, your symptoms will become more prominent and demand your attention.

Looking after yourself, I believe, starts with understanding how you deserve to nourish and care for yourself. This encompasses the physical aspects of your life as well as the emotional. That means taking the time to instil good sleep habits, eat nourishing foods, foster positive relationships and rest.

I've learned the hard way over the years that I need time to myself in order to function in life, to support my family and maintain standards in my work. If I don't take this time, I tend to reach a critical point where I'm exhausted, irritable and highly anxious, sleeping poorly and unable to concentrate. So I save up and, when feasible, I rent a place in rural Ireland for a few days on my own, where I hike, read and watch boxsets – I do everything on my own schedule, sleeping and rising when I like (if I want to stay in bed and read until lunchtime, then I do; if I feel like some air at 6 a.m., I go for a walk), and cooking and eating whatever I want whenever I feel like it. It's a huge reset for me, and the feeling of freedom when I get in the car and set off for an adventure is elating. When I was younger, I would have been quite worried about doing things like this on my own, but the need to look after myself has become stronger than my anxiety, and it's something I look forward to hugely. Even the planning feels calming and rejuvenating – a little space just for me.

– Hannah

WHO AM I NOW?

Women who commit themselves to family life, their career, or their partner's job sometimes begin to feel robbed, undervalued and as if their lives have not been lived on their terms. The energy invested in their family or their career has the potential to become their identity. What happens when they lose their role in their family and their children start to leave home, or if they lose their job? They may begin to feel trapped, anxious, and lose their sense of self. 'Who am I now?' they may wonder. Midlife can be a good moment to re-evaluate this, and a renewed sense of your potential can emerge.

It may be that you are sandwiched between many responsibilities, with growing children, ageing parents, work and life in general all coming together at the same junction as menopause. It can be chaotic; it can be overwhelming. Taking time to rest and restore is essential. These are the years to ask for help – at home with family members; at work with your manager and colleagues. We all need support to thrive through menopause. Sadly, sometimes we are not very good at asking for it. I would encourage you to grab a sheet of paper, list those aspects that you feel are tipping you over the edge, and see where and how you can build in more support.

THE MINDSET OF MENOPAUSE

Do you like change? Do you believe that menopause is a natural change of life? As humans, we don't tend to automatically love change, yet it is a part of everyday life. Change can be tough, but nearly always it is worth it. Menopause comes with a heightened change. It's asking you to dig deep and embrace the changes that are happening on all levels for you to emerge into a stronger, more confident, freer version of you. Taking an informed, empowered view of menopause will help you adopt a positive growth mindset toward it. I know this can be hard, particularly as we often hear fearful stories of menopause in the media. I hope the practical tools and options throughout this book will help you know that you have many resources to draw on and that your menopause years are to be embraced for the new chapter in your life they bring.

Below are some things to consider when it comes to minding yourself in these years.

JOURNALING

I have a large selection of journals – every holiday I return with a new one. I love writing; I love the physical process of getting thoughts onto paper. Journaling is a private space to work out any issues you may be facing or offload some emotions you are feeling. In *The Artist's Way*, Julia Cameron recommends a brain dump every day, to just let your mind flow, writing whatever comes into it. I cannot recommend this enough. It is the best form of free therapy you will ever get (apart from sleep!). There is no right or wrong way to journal – it's simply writing anything you want and it can relate to any aspect of your life. If possible, use the physical form of writing – pen and paper: this way you are putting new ideas into your subconscious mind more effectively than typing on a laptop or phone.

GRATITUDE

Being grateful helps us to pause and reflect on the present moment and the positive aspects of our existence. Even on terrible days, there is always something to be grateful for. Some days may be more difficult than others, but pausing to reflect is extremely beneficial for keeping life in perspective. When you're in the grip of anxiety, this can be a modest stepping stone to help you go forward and see the light at the end of the tunnel.

Robert Emmons, the world's leading scientific authority on gratitude, has detailed the benefits of everyday appreciation, which include more restful sleep, increased immune system performance and reduced blood pressure – and that's just the beginning. That should be enough motivation to take a few minutes each morning and evening to be grateful.

I keep a gratitude journal and write in it every day – it could be minor details or major life events. I usually do it in the evening as part of my night-time routine, and I always feel lighter and calmer after it. It's another one of those habits that you won't regret, so go out and purchase a lovely notebook and get started. Personally, I like to write by hand, but there are apps available if that is more convenient for you.

MULTITASKING IS NOT YOUR FRIEND

I used to think I was doing great by combining different activities and tasks – as women, we push ourselves to do this. Now we know this isn't the case, and multitasking is no friend to your brain health and certainly not in your menopause years. Concentrating on one single task at a time is critical. Your concentration will be solely focused, your productivity will be better, as you are being completely present to the job at hand, and you will feel calmer.

ROUTINE

Finding and establishing a habit or routine that works for you is a great way of minding yourself. You can develop a self-care regimen to energise, spark and nurture your mind, body and soul, whatever your daily role in life. As humans we love routine; it anchors us to life. How you start your day is part of this. Jay Shetty, in *Think Like a Monk*, refers to the morning 'mental shower' he has, where he practises meditation and downtime before the day starts. Early rising can be part of your morning routine – that time of the day when the house and the world are quieter is my favourite time. If you start getting up earlier, make sure you use that time for yourself. Don't get into household chores: use it to read, meditate, journal, have a cup of tea, whatever makes you smile. Take time – don't speed through your life.

A good idea here is to plan your morning the night before. So for me, I leave my clothes out, a book I will read a few pages of and anything else that fits my routine. The night before sets the scene.

BOUNDARIES

Boundaries are powerful. You can maintain your self-respect and energy, and also protect your time, through them. As you go through life and menopause, they are a necessity. We often struggle with maintaining healthy boundaries, and this can become an added stress during your menopause. Menopause wants us to have concrete-like boundaries. It wants us to be able to say no, firmly and with power, and put a focus on ourselves when needed. Establishing healthy boundaries can be uncomfortable – you are asking people who have established relationships with you to change how they treat you. But this is you respecting yourself. If you don't, you may say yes to everything and become overwhelmed by responsibilities. Setting boundaries is similar to putting a perimeter around yourself and determining what is and is not appropriate for you. Learn to say no: it will protect you from being burnt out and leave you with time to mind yourself.

If this is an area you feel you can work on, see Resources for more.

I take supplements – vitamins C, D, omegas, B complex, calcium and magnesium. I make sure my diet gives me what I need and I do yoga, walking and weight-bearing exercise. I also meditate and I do breath work to keep my mind calm and energised. I feel good now. I am very grateful my symptoms are mild and I am really listening to my body more than I ever have before. I feel this time has brought a deeper understanding of my body and given it the time and attention it deserves.

– Georgina

DOWNTIME FROM TECHNOLOGY

One of the advantages of being in our forties and fifties is that we didn't grow up immersed in the virtual environment of social media – it's taxing. Unfortunately, our lives are on display to a level that has never been seen before, and our brains may not have fully developed to deal with the stress this puts us under on a regular basis.

There are undeniably positive parts to social media, ranging from fantastic recipes to advice, not to mention the chance to communicate with many more people than you could in the physical world. However, I believe it should come with cautions, such as restricting your time, avoiding addiction and reminding yourself of the superficiality of a filtered world where hardly anyone publishes a bad photo and and many people feel unrestrained in the opinions they express.

Our brains also require quiet downtime in order to be rejuvenated, resilient and capable of dealing with daily life events. So I recommend doing a daily digital detox – start by putting your phone away for an hour at a time that is convenient for you. You'll notice how much more comfortable you are without the continual pings or the need to check it. It will help you to disconnect and be present. Even better is to turn off notifications. Or to start your day by not going straight to the phone – give yourself an hour or two before turning it on. Another great step is to establish one technology-free day each week.

BE GENTLE AND KIND TO YOURSELF

It took a long time for Rome to be built. To get a handle on your menopause, you'll need knowledge, time and thoughtfulness. Go slowly, make tiny improvements, and don't try to accomplish too much at once. We know from James Clear's *Atomic Habits* that making minor tweaks to established habits is a more effective strategy to make long-term changes.

Perhaps we should start by, above all, being kind and compassionate to ourselves.

Part 5: What's Next?

23

Opening up – a chapter for your partner

I have met many supportive partners over the years – the husbands who bought tickets for their wives to attend events I held, the partners who emailed me when both were going through menopause, the husband fearing for his wife's mental health, the wife whose menopause was a breeze compared to her partner's. So many stories! The uniting aspect of all was love and feeling at a loss for what to do.

All the self-help books on relationships will tell you how important communication is, and now, in menopause, there is no getting away from this. Communication, compassion and understanding are key.

This chapter is for partners – to explain a little of what is going on, the changes that might be happening and how to offer support. If you are going through menopause, please hand this book to your nearest and dearest and ask them, at a minimum, to read this chapter. If you are the partner of someone going through it, then the rest of this is for you – your understanding, concern and support could make all the difference.

HOW TO SUPPORT SOMEONE GOING THROUGH MENOPAUSE

Education

Before you even start the conversation with your partner about what she is experiencing, read up and try to understand what menopause is all about. A great place to start is this book in your hands. Menopause is so much more than society believes it to be. Learning about it will help you maintain compassionate relationships with those in your life going through it. It will help you understand why maybe she gets cross with you, why she may be feeling low and just not herself at the moment. You'll even feel better, as you will understand that it's not about you: it's the hormonal upheaval that's happening. She needs not only your support but also your understanding now more than ever. Remember: this is a chapter and it will close.

Opening the conversation

It's possible you're reading this before your partner, that you've seen changes and signs she doesn't seem to be aware of, and you'd like to talk to her about it. Many partners send links to blogs or podcasts in an attempt to start the conversation, and this is one way to approach it. Just be mindful that if the perimenopausal person in your life is in denial and unaware of what is happening, this may not be the best approach. It is certainly worth a try, but I think talking face to face or side by side with someone is a better first step, as you can see their reaction and you will be better able to judge if you are on the right route. If you feel you hit a wall with talking, then maybe print out a gentle introduction to menopause and suggest they could talk to their doctor and get things checked out. You could make the nudge gently, direct them to a website, mention something on the radio – a small hint can start this important conversation.

A listening ear

The floodgates may not open initially, but eventually they will. Be ready. Just listen – don't judge. Have your ears and mind totally open. We all know how powerful it is when we are listened to and how bad we feel when we aren't. So drop everything (within reason) and be there. Ask how you can help, and be ready and willing to deliver on anything you promise. It won't help if you commit to something and don't follow through.

> One thing I have learnt about menopause is that you can't fix it, and your relationship shifts or changes its dynamic. When my wife talks about menopause I used to jump into 'what can I do' mode. How can I fix it? Now I know it's all about listening and having my ears open. Making the cup of tea at night-time goes down very well too!'
>
> – Pat

The power of kindness

My dad used to always say 'be kind', among many other things. I like to think it's a characteristic of the years he was with us. We all respond to kindness, even if it is with a somewhat bitter acknowledgement, tears or a smile. All humans respond to acts of kindness. You can do these regularly – those small gestures will have great meaning in menopause. Making a cup of tea, cooking the dinner, doing the shopping, suggesting a walk outside – these simple acts can mean a lot to someone who is overwhelmed due to sleep issues and other menopausal symptoms. You will know what the woman in your life enjoys and what will relieve some pressure from her day.

Don't take it personally

Introspection, desiring peace and quiet, not being talkative and avoiding social occasions can be a part of these years. In my early perimenopause years I wanted to hibernate and just find somewhere quiet away from the world. As a partner, you might struggle with this and think it's you: it's not. Thousands of women report that need to be alone, to take stock. Helping your partner get the balance right is key, as it isn't helpful for them to withdraw too much – we all need support through life.

But when the quiet times hit, don't take it personally. Offer gentle support and know that it's another stage of the process.

Last-minute changes

Social anxiety and exhaustion are very common in menopause. For many women, going out and having to be social can be a step too far. For most, this is temporary, but it can still last for some time. Be supportive and aware that often being in the comfort and security of your home may be more attractive than a night out. The majority of the time this is due to loss of confidence, anxiety and exhaustion. We all feel our most secure at home with those we love and trust, especially at the end of a busy week at work.

The stormy moods

They will happen: there will be tense moments, possibly unkind words. If you can, remember what is happening and cut your partner a little slack. However, do honour yourself too. If it becomes too much, then you must encourage outside help and support. It is important to remember menopause impacts not only the person going through it but also you as a partner, and your partner also needs to acknowledge what she is going through.

Talk about sex

Many people find this the hardest aspect of menopause to discuss with those close to them, yet it is arguably the most important. Both of you may feel unloved and no longer attractive if there is no communication in relation to your sexual health as a couple. I have met many women who felt so sad that this aspect of their lives had stopped. They felt they had lost the connection and intimacy with their partners that they had enjoyed for many years.

If sexual activity is not happening, I would encourage you not to take this personally. Consider reading Chapter 6, as this will offer insight into what is happening in relation to libido and sexual health. Ongoing acts of kindness and thoughtfulness will help here, as libido and arousal change as we age and women, for the majority, don't tend to get aroused as quickly as they once did. That's why the overall relationship is fundamental.

To keep sex a part of your life, it may mean your partner obtaining medical advice or introducing things that weren't an aspect of your sexual life before – be kind and understand that your partner may feel awkward in doing this. And try to be open to it – it just might start a new chapter of exploration and increased intimacy in your relationship.

Talk to each other

This sounds easy, right? But it's not. Emotions and feelings often get in the way and can make things even more difficult as your partner goes through menopause. Being able to talk openly is the foundation of a healthy relationship and an essential part of the journey of menopause. You can start this conversation gently by asking how your partner is feeling and how you can help. The more chats you have, the more you will both learn and the better you can support each other.

Encourage outside help

Many partners have contacted me to ask where and how they can get support for those they love who are struggling and afraid. The first place to start is with a good GP. Maybe offer to go to the appointment as well – you can sit in or stay outside. If brain fog and anxiety are issues, your partner may struggle to remember and articulate what she is feeling. Your support here can be of great benefit to you both.

Your relationship

Unfortunately, many couples separate during these years. There, of course, may be valid reasons for this not pertaining to menopause, but menopause can be a factor. Supporting your partner through menopause will only reinforce your relationship if this is an issue.

* * *

Your partner may breeze through menopause, but given that 75 per cent of women experience some of the symptoms, you will probably see some changes through these years. Often you may notice them before she does. Being supportive and showing kindness will change the experience for both of you.

24

Shattering the taboo in a diverse and inclusive way

Menopause requires support across all society. The many and varied conversations we are having all lead to the same end goal: menopause education for everyone and supporting all who experience menopause. I have been privileged to work with people experiencing many forms of menopause – andropause (male menopause), natural menopause, early menopause – and some who are experiencing these while living with a disability or facing discrimination. Sadly, we know and see daily the health inequality that exists in relation to many aspects of life and menopause in particular. Having worked with women with Down syndrome and intellectual disabilities and those facing daily racial discrimination, I have seen first-hand the harsh realities and additional challenges they face while navigating menopause.

Do you remember your mum speaking about menopause? I certainly don't, but I do remember my mum being hot and flustered in the kitchen over Sunday roasts. Menopause wasn't spoken about – the taboo and shame was strong.

HOW DO WE SHATTER THE TABOO?

We change. We evolve. We talk. Every conversation is a stepping stone to change.

Today we talk more openly about periods, and the term 'period power' is becoming more acceptable within society. Menopause is on the same journey. It is becoming acceptable to use the word, to discuss this sensitive time in a person's life. We need this. When a woman is struggling at work due to symptoms, she should be able to express what is happening and take time off when symptoms are challenging and impacting her day without being judged unable to perform her job. We do a disservice to so many by not supporting each other through all aspects of menopause in our daily lives. Many women go part-time at work because their symptoms dictate their lives. This is fine if you're happy to do it, but it is far from fine if you want to continue in your role and advance in your career.

Menopause demands that you rest. It wants you to slow down, sit with the changes that are happening and evolve into the new you. This is difficult in society and a struggle to balance with our daily lives.

WHERE DOES CHANGE START?

We can change the approach to menopause with education and information:

Menopause in the health-care system: education for all families; education for minority groups – for example, women with intellectual disabilities, women in the Travelling community, women from marginalised parts of society; education around the choices available to women – lifestyle changes, medical interventions and so on; enhanced education and awareness for GPs in relation to menopause.

Early menopause: enhanced support for POI, early menopause and surgical menopause/medically induced menopause.

Menopause in the workplace: promoting awareness in the workplace of the symptoms of menopause and ensuring in-house support. Women can be at their most creative in menopause – this needs to be embraced and women acknowledged for the knowledge and wisdom they have gained over the years.

Secondary school education: the addition of menopause to the curriculum. The UK has achieved this, and all countries should follow suit.

In October 2022 the Irish government took a global lead by launching the first national menopause awareness campaign. This was a momentous step in changing attitudes across society. In addition, a new national online resource for menopause was launched, offering the first go-to point in Ireland. (See Resources.)

Menopause is inevitable for all women – this part of life cannot be bypassed. Society needs to embrace it as much as other life events. How society views menopause will impact how a woman experiences it. The Western view of ageing is not as accepting as it should be – we need to change this. We need to abandon negative thoughts about ageing and embrace this process, defy the culture of ageism and instead revere women for the wisdom and authenticity menopause brings. This is liberation.

RACIAL AND CULTURAL VARIATIONS

Cultural variations exist when it comes to menopause; your way of life and traditions will all have a role to play. Add to this varying diets, exercise regimes, attitudes to ageing and your own and society's attitudes to menopause – all these influence how you transition through these years and experience symptoms.

The SWAN study shows that Black and Latina women experience menopause at a younger age (average forty-eight years) and also more severely. Black women experience more fibroids, are at increased risk of hysterectomy, have more skin and hair issues and tend not to openly discuss menopause. Stress and socioeconomic status also impact a woman's experience, and for many ethnic groups, racial discrimination is sadly an added stress to be borne.

We know that the Traveller and Roma communities experience discrimination across society, and the challenges women in these communities face are compounded as they move into menopause, especially in relation to the emotional and psychological aspects of those years.

In Turkey and among Muslim women, menopause is often seen as 'unclean', 'the curse of Allah', and shame shrouds these years. In India, there is a general negative view of all things menstrual, which compounds women's difficulties in the menopause transition.

On a positive note, Japanese women are some of the healthiest in the world and live five years longer, on average, than women in the West. They have lower rates of osteoporosis, breast cancer and heart disease. Cultural and environmental factors have a big role to play here. We also see different symptoms, with chilliness being experienced by more women in Japan than hot flushes, and shoulder pain being very common. Their diet, which is high in soy isoflavones, is a major health benefit. So the symptoms of menopause are not universally experienced.

Attitudes to the matriarchal role in the community differ around the world. Native American and Indigenous Australian cultures both state an increased level of respect when menopause is reached. These women are (rightly) considered within the community as 'women of wisdom'. Mayan women celebrate when they hit menopause – it is seen as a freedom and reaching the pinnacle in their communities as spiritual leaders. Mayan women report the earliest age for natural menopause as 44.3 years. This is thought to be because they spend so many years in a reproductive or postnatal state, which means low oestrogen supplies in the body. They also live in communities where the menstrual cycle comes with strict rules, so the cessation of periods is a very freeing and welcomed event.

LEARNING DISABILITIES

Menopause is complex and there is a lot of information to absorb. This presents additional challenges when you have a learning disability. From my experience, many such women have been totally unprepared for menopause and had no idea what would happen in their bodies. Menopause can occur earlier for those with Down syndrome and those with a history of seizures.

Lack of information and support means women are not aware of the symptoms and also the possible treatment options. Education of all women, including their carers, is key here, and it needs to be approached in the right way – stories, pictures and objects can make it easier for those with learning difficulties to grasp what is happening and be supported to ask for help when needed and not feel isolated. HRT can be tricky, as many may not welcome the daily prescription or application, and sadly their symptoms are often not taken seriously by doctors. This is an area that needs change fast and one where we are failing women.

NEURODIVERSITY

To date research is limited but it tells us that ADHD, ASD and other types of neurodiversity can result in heightened menopause symptoms, especially in relation to the psychological aspect. It can be hard to distinguish menopause symptoms from certain ASD or ADHD symptoms, and these tend to be worse in the early perimenopause years as oestrogen fluctuates.

GENDER

People of all gender identities may experience menopause or menopause symptoms. As gender is a spectrum, every individual experience must be listened to. Research is very lacking in this area and little direction is given. This needs to change, as so many additional challenges exist for people transitioning through menopause on this spectrum. A 2011 US survey showed that 19 per cent of transgender or gender non-conforming people were refused medical treatment on the grounds of discrimination, with 50 per cent having to inform their medical advisors of what they needed. The additional medical checks and investigations through the menopause years may cause added distress and anxiety. All of this is compounded, too, by the increased risk of social marginalisation, isolation, past and present trauma, discrimination and depression. Trans health is a growing field and much more research and compassion is needed. A step in the right direction is the proposed change to the NICE guidelines in the UK to include trans and non-binary people.

FINANCIAL COST

Menopause has become big business globally, and I would encourage you to take a symptom-by-symptom approach when investing in new services or products. Determine what is essential and what will support *you* personally. The aim of the 6 Ms is to offer practical, inexpensive support as you navigate these years. In an ideal world, many menopause-related services would be publicly funded, but we have some work to do yet in that area. The sometimes rocky road of menopause should not be made more difficult because of financial concerns.

MY INVITATION TO YOU

I invite you to consider the potential these years can bring to you and be open to new pathways and changes that can enter your life. Menopause should not be a dark chapter in a woman's life. With knowledge and support, this is a chapter in which to thrive, renew and embrace a whole new you.

It will happen by educating and supporting women, their partners and their families in knowing and understanding menopause and the uniqueness of this time for every woman. Our generation is already experiencing a different menopause from our parents. The next generation will have a totally different experience – my three sons talk about menopause like it's just another simple part of life. Ireland has achieved many great steps forward, and there is plenty of room for more.

This is my vision for the future: it starts in the home and in school, learning about menopause in secondary school; talking about it openly at home; when you are forty-five (for natural menopause), you receive a reminder for your perimenopause check with your local GP or community health centre. This check makes sure you are aware of all the symptoms of menopause – the good, the bad and the ugly. It prepares you for what might happen in your body. It alerts you to the red flags. You know what your treatment options are, from HRT to non-hormonal to complementary therapies. You can make informed choices. Along with this, you have a free check with a women's-health physiotherapist to see how things are going in the core and urinary side and, yes, for vaginal dryness and pelvic prolapse too. Then you are booked in for a bone-density (DXA) scan. You are fully informed; you are fully aware of the symptoms of menopause and so are those around you. The taboo is shattered across society.

How you transition through these years is important. It impacts your future. Your menopause years will have a direct effect on how you age, offering you a unique opportunity to future-proof your body for optimum health in the years ahead.

Menopause is much more than hot flushes and brain fog. It is a deeply psychological path to a new you. While it can look like it is happening externally and physically, it really is an internal, exclusive change that happens to you – no other person will experience it as you do.

Cycles of life are embedded deeply in our being – nature in all its beauty, the cycle of the moon and oceans, the seasons, our menstrual cycles. Constant change, creation and the cyclical nature of our lives is manifested throughout. Menopause offers you the opportunity to renew, reclaim your inner power and become your true self. For many, it is a time of monumental growth and potential.

The journey of menopause, of coming home, has one constant: change. With all the fluctuating hormones, your body is literally transforming internally. And for many, change comes with emotional upheaval and pain.

Menopause is a process and it is not always easy or fun. Far from it. It can be chaotic, complicated, complex, embarrassing and clumsy. It may be the biggest challenge you have yet encountered – and all the while, you have to go about your day-to-day life. You have to work, to juggle, to support others.

But it is a transformation. A liberation. It is, as the Japanese say, *konenki* – a time of renewal and energy. Menopause is a time to slow down and and allow your body to gently adjust to a new status quo. To take time for you. To show yourself what you show everyone else: kindness. Menopause encourages you to be your happy and whole self.

If you reach menopause at the age of fifty, you may be only a little more than halfway through your life – and many will say that the second part is the better part. Menopause and ageing don't have to take the pleasure out of life: incorporating the practical steps outlined in these pages can help ease symptoms, future-proof your health, promote longevity and allow you to thrive.

It's your menopause, no one else's, and you don't have to suffer in silence. We can support each other, take time to look after ourselves and shatter the taboo of menopause for good.

Resources

General

Catherine O'Keeffe, Wellness Warrior:
wellnesswarrior.ie

Irish Department of Health: gov.ie/menopause

Menopause Support: menopausesupport.co.uk

Women's Health Concern: womens-health-concern.org

2. When menopause comes early

ARC Cancer Support Centres: arccancersupport.ie

Daisy Network: daisynetwork.org

Daisy Network: Our Guide to Understanding Premature Ovarian Insufficiency. Tolworth: Grosvenor House Publishing, 2021.

Dr Hannah Short and Dr Mandy Leonhardt. *The Complete Guide to POI and Early Menopause.* London: Sheldon Press, 2022.

European Society of Human Reproduction and Embryology: eshre.eu

Irish Cancer Society: cancer.ie

Marie Keating Foundation: mariekeating.ie

3. Symptoms – an overview

fibroireland.com

The Irish Nutrition and Dietetic Institute: indi.ie

Migraine Ireland: migraine.ie

Nutritional Therapists of Ireland: ntoi.ie

4. Sleep

https://cbti.ie

5. Genitourinary symptoms of menopause

Constipation: squattypotty.eu

Continence Foundation of Ireland: Continence.ie

iscp.ie/ (select women's health under Find a Physio)

Overactive bladder: OAB.ie

Pelvic floor exercises:
pelvicfloorfirst.org.au
pelvicexercises.com.au

Pelvic physiotherapy: pelvicphysiotherapy.com

Support sportswear: evbsport.com

Vaginal moisturisers and lubricants:
Yes Organics – yesyesyes.org
Olive and Bee – oliveandbee.com.au

6. Let's talk about sex

Accredited psychosexual and relationship therapists: sextherapists.ie

Sex toys:
jodivine.com
sexsiopa.ie

7. Bone health

Irish Osteoporosis Society:
www.irishosteoporosis.ie

mindyourbones.ie/

Royal Osteoporosis Society: theros.org.uk

8. Maintaining a healthy brain

Alzheimer Society of Ireland: alzheimer.ie

Dr Lisa Mosconi: lisamosconi.com

11. Minding your heart

Alcohol: hse.ie/alcohol

Croí: croi.ie

Irish Heart Foundation: irishheart.ie

Smoking: hse.ie/quit-smoking

Stress: stresscontrol.ie

12. The psychological side of menopause

Babette Rothschild. *The Body Remembers: The Psychophysiology of Trauma and Trauma Treatment.* W. W. Norton, 2000.

Bessel van der Kolk. *The Body Keeps the Score: Mind, Brain and Body in the Transformation of Trauma.* Penguin, 2014.

CBT:
CBT for menopausal symptoms: womens-health-concern.org/help-and-advice/factsheets/cognitive-behaviour-therapy-cbt-menopausal-symptoms/

Trauma-focused CBT: tfcbt.org

Pamela Myles-Hooton. *The CBT Handbook*. Robinson Press, 2015.

EMDR (Eye Movement Desensitisation and Reprocessing) All-Ireland Association: emdrireland.org

Mental Health Ireland: mentalhealthireland.ie

Rape Crisis Network Ireland: rcni.ie

Rewind technique for dealing with PTSD and trauma: hgi.org.uk/useful-information/treatment-dealing-ptsd-trauma-phobias/rewind-technique

Suicide prevention and support: 3ts.ie

13. Menopause at work

citizensinformationboard.ie

wellnesswarrior.ie/workplace

14. Uncovering HRT

HRT: hse.ie/conditions/hrt

National Institute for Health and Care Excellence: nice.org.uk/guidance/ng23

womens-health-concern.org

15. Other treatments

acupuncturecouncilofireland.com

Breath of Life Natural Healing Clinic: bolhealing.com

Essential oils:

thenatureofthings.ie

kotanical.ie

atlanticaromatics.com

floraplusfiona.com

irishhomeopathy.ie

Irish Register of Herbalists: irh.ie

osteopathy.ie

reflexology.ie

reikifederationireland.com

17. MOT – your menopause check-in

irishdermatologists.ie

iscp.ie/ (select women's health under Find a Physio)

National Institute for Health and Care Excellence: nice.org.uk/guidance/ng23

19. Menu – the importance of food

The Irish Nutrition and Dietetic Institute: indi.ie.

Nutritional Therapists of Ireland: ntoi.ie

22. Minding you – crucial care

Nedra Glover Tawwab. *Set Boundaries, Find Peace*. New York: Penguin, 2021.

23. Shattering the taboo in a diverse and inclusive way

Government of Ireland menopause website: gov.ie/en/campaigns/menopause/?referrer=http://www.gov.ie/menopause/.

MENOPAUSE SYMPTOM CHECKER

SYMPTOM	YES	NO	DETAILS
PSYCHOLOGICAL			
Anxiety			
Low mood			
Depression			
Mood swings			
Crying spells			
Brain fog			
Loss of confidence			
Poor concentration			
Poor memory			
Loss of joy			
Reduced self-esteem			
Irritability			
Palpitations			
Panic attacks			
Difficulty sleeping			
Tired/lacking energy			
PHYSICAL			
Headaches			
Migraines			
Painful/aching joints			
Restless leg syndrome			
Hot flushes			
Night sweats			
Cold sweats			
Changes to periods			
PMT-like symptoms			
Digestive issues			
Painful sex			
Loss of libido			

SYMPTOM	YES	NO	DETAILS
Electric shock			
Feeling dizzy/faint			
Dry eyes/ears/mouth			
Oral health changes			
Thinning hair			
Dry/itchy skin (formication)			
Tinnitus			
Restless legs			
Change to body odour			
Increased allergies			
Histamine intolerance			
GENITOURINARY			
Vaginal/vulval dryness			
Vaginal/vulval soreness			
Vaginal/vulval irritation			
Vaginal/vulval pain			
Vaginal/vulval burning			
Skin thinning or splitting			
Labia shrinking			
Clitoral shrinking/pain			
Watery discharge			
Painful episiotomy scar			
Abnormal vaginal bleeding			
Bleeding after intercourse			
Repeated urinary infections			
Urge urinary incontinence			
Stress incontinence			
Pelvic organ prolapse			
Painful smear test			

Symptom checkers are available to download from
wellnesswarrior.ie and menopausesupport.co.uk

Bibliography

Adetunji, Jo. 'The brain also produces the sex hormone oestrogen.' 13 December 2013. theconversation.com. Accessed 15 August 2022.

AlAwlaqi, Ahmed and Mohamed Hammadeh. 'Examining the relationship between hormone therapy and dry-eye syndrome in postmenopausal women: a cross-sectional comparison study.' *Menopause* 23, no. 5 (2016): 550–5.

Ali, Siti Atiyah, Tahamina Begum and Faruque Reza. 'Hormonal influences on cognitive function.' *The Malaysian Journal of Medical Sciences: MJMS* 25, no. 4 (2018): 31–41.

Allen, Andrew P. and Andrew P. Smith. 'Chewing gum: cognitive performance, mood, well-being, and associated physiology.' *BioMed Research International 2015* (2015): 654806.

Alzheimer's Association Report. '2020 Alzheimer's disease facts and figures.' *Alzheimer's & Dementia* 16 (2020): 391–460.

American Cancer Society. 'Endometrial cancer risk factors.' cancer.org. Accessed 5 August 2022.

American Chemical Society. 'Russell Marker and the Mexican steroid hormone industry.' October 1999. acs.org. Accessed 12 August 2022.

Anderson, Scott C. *et al.* The *Psychobiotic Revolution*. Washington DC: National Geographic Partners, 2017.

Anjum, Ibrar *et al.* 'The role of vitamin D in brain health: a mini literature review.' *Cureus* 10, no. 7 (2018): e2960.

Association of UK Dietitians, 'Probiotics and gut health: Food Fact Sheet', bda.uk.com. Accessed 30 October 2022.

Australian Menopause Society. 'Bioidentical hormones for menopausal symptoms.' January 2007. imsociety.org. Accessed 12 August 2022.

Australian Menopause Society. 'Menopause – combined hormone (replacement therapy).' September 2004. imsociety.org. Accessed 12 August 2022.

Australian Menopause Society. 'Treating the menopause – the concept of risk and benefit.' August 2008. imsociety.org. Accessed 12 August 2022.

Avis, Nancy E. and Sybil Crawford. 'Cultural differences in symptoms and attitudes toward menopause.' menopausemgmt.com. 21 September 2007. Accessed 28 July 2022.

Avis, Nancy E. *et al.* 'Acupuncture in menopause (AIM) study: a pragmatic, randomized controlled trial.' *Menopause* 23, no. 6 (2016): 626–37.

Baber, R.J., N. Panay, A. Fenton, the IMS Writing Group. '2016 IMS recommendations on women's midlife health and menopause hormone therapy.' *Climacteric* 19, no. 2 (2016): 109–50.

Bansal, Ramandeep and Neelam Aggarwal. 'Menopausal hot flashes: a concise review.' *Journal of Midlife Health* 10, no. 1 (2019): 6–13.

'Barbiturate abuse.' webmd.com. Accessed 12 August 2022.

Baulieu E., M. Schumacher. 'Progesterone as a neuroactive neurosteroid, with special reference to the effect of progesterone on myelination.' *Steroids* 65, no. 10–11 (2000): 605–12.

Beall, C.M. 'Ages at menopause and menarche in a high-altitude Himalayan population.' *Annals of Human Biology* 10, no. 4 (1983): 365–70.

Benshushan, Abraham *et al.* 'IUD use and the risk of endometrial cancer.' *European Journal of Obstetrics, Gynecology, and Reproductive Biology* 105, no. 2 (2002): 166–9.

Beral, Valerie *et al.* 'Ovarian cancer and hormone replacement therapy in the Million Women Study.' *Lancet* 369, no. 9574 (2007): 1703–10.

Berger, Julian Meyer *et al.* 'Mediation of the acute stress response by the skeleton.' *Cell Metabolism* 30, no. 5 (2019): 890–902.

Berin, Emilia *et al*. 'Resistance training for
hot flushes in postmenopausal women: a
randomised controlled trial.' *Maturitas* 126
(2019): 55–60.

Bjelland Elisabeth. K. *et al*. 'The relation of age
at menarche with age at natural menopause:
a population study of 336,788 women in
Norway.' *Human Reproduction* 33, no. 6 (2018):
1149–57.

Bódis, J., H.R. Tinneberg, A. Török *et al*. 'Effect of
noradrenaline and dopamine on progesterone
and estradiol secretion of human granulosa
cells.' *Acta Endocrinologica* 129, no. 2 (1993):
165–68.

Bódis, J., H.R. Tinneberg, H. Schwarz *et al*.
'The effect of histamine on progesterone and
estradiol secretion of human granulosa cells in
serum-free culture.' *Gynecological Endocrinology*
7, no. 4 (1993): 235–9.

Bojar, Iwona *et al*. 'Postmenopausal cognitive
changes and androgen levels in the context
of apolipoprotein E polymorphism.' *Archives
of Medical Science*: AMS 13, no. 5 (2017):
1148–1159.

Bordet, M.F. *et al*. 'Treating hot flushes in
menopausal women with homeopathic
treatment – results of an observational
study.' Homeopathy: *The Journal of the Faculty
of Homeopathy* 97, no. 1 (2008): 10–5.

Briden, Lara. *Hormone Repair Manual*. Greenpeak,
2021.

Brinton, Roberta D. *et al*. 'Perimenopause as a
neurological transition state.' *Nature Reviews
Endocrinology* 11, no. 7 (2015): 393–405.

British Menopause Society. 'What are the
alternative treatment options to HRT?'
thebms.org.uk. Accessed 10 August 2022.

Brodhead, Havilah. 'The ups and downs of
bioidentical hormones: everything you should
know.' 23 June 2021. hearthsidemedicine.com.
Accessed 12 August 2022.

Bromberger, Joyce T. and Howard M. Kravitz.
'Mood and menopause: findings from the
Study of Women's Health Across the Nation
(SWAN) over 10 years.' *Obstetrics and*

Gynecology Clinics of North America 38, no. 3
(2011): 609–25.

'Carbamazepine – uses, side effects, and more.'
webmd.com. Accessed 12 August 2022.

'Carbamazepine.' nhs.uk. Accessed 12 August
2022.

Carmody, James Francis *et al*. 'Mindfulness
training for coping with hot flashes: results of a
randomized trial.' *Menopause* 18, no. 6 (2011):
611–20.

Carrasquilla, Germán D. *et al*. 'Postmenopausal
hormone therapy and risk of stroke: a pooled
analysis of data from population-based cohort
studies.' *PLOS Medicine* 14, no. 11 (2017):
e1002445.

Celec, Peter, Daniela Ostatníková and Július
Hodosy. 'On the effects of testosterone on
brain behavioral functions.' *Frontiers in
Neuroscience* 9, no. 12. (2015).

Centers for Disease Control. 'Leading causes
of death – females – all races and origins
– United States, 2017.' cdc.gov. Accessed 5
August 2022.

Centre for Menstrual Cycle and Ovulation
Research. 'Perimenopause.' cemcor.ubc.ca.
Accessed 5 August 2022.

Chen, Li-Ru, Nai-Yu Ko and Kuo-Hu Chen.
'Isoflavone supplements for menopausal
women: a systematic review.' *Nutrients* 11, no.
11 (2019): 2649.

Clear, James. *Atomic Habits*. London: Penguin,
2018.

Cohen, Lee S. *et al*. 'Risk for new onset
of depression during the menopausal
transition: the Harvard study of moods and
cycles.' *Archives of General Psychiatry* 63, no. 4
(2006): 385–90.

Columbia University Irving Medical Center.
'Bone, not adrenaline drives fight or flight
response.' 12 September 2019. cuimc.columbia.
edu. Accessed 15 August 2022.

'Common sleep disorders.' my.clevelandclinic.org.
Accessed 17 August 2022.

Cramer, Holger, Wenbo Peng and Romy Lauche.
'Yoga for menopausal symptoms: a systematic

review and meta-analysis.' *Maturitas* 109 (2018): 13–25.

Curhan, Sharon G. *et al.* 'Menopause and postmenopausal hormone therapy and risk of hearing loss.' *Menopause (New York, N.Y.)* 24, no. 9 (2017): 1049–56.

Currie, Heather. 'Menopause and insomnia.' September 2021. womens-health-concern.org. Accessed 17 August 2022.

Cylwik, Bogdan *et al.* 'Vitamin B12 concentration in the blood of alcoholics.' *Polski merkuriusz lekarski: organ Polskiego Towarzystwa Lekarskiego* 28, no. 164 (2010): 122–5.

Daley, Amanda *et al.* 'Exercise for vasomotor menopausal symptoms.' *The Cochrane Database of Systematic Reviews*, 11 (2014): CD006108.

Dana, Deb. *The Polyvagal Theory in Therapy*. New York: Norton Professional Books, 2018.

De Villiers, T.J. and S.R. Goldstein. 'Update on bone health: the International Menopause Society white paper 2021.' September 2021. imsociety.org. Accessed 12 August 2022.

Dean, Carolyn. *The Magnesium Miracle*. New York: Ballantine Books, 2017.

'Design of the Women's Health Initiative clinical trial and observational study. The Women's Health Initiative Study Group.' *Controlled Clinical Trials* 19, no. 1 (1998): 61–109.

Diabetes Ireland. 'Diabetes prevalence in Ireland.' January 2022. diabetes.ie. Accessed 15 August 2022.

Diabetes Ireland. 'Get sugar smart.' diabetes.ie. Accessed 15 August 2022.

DiNicolantonio, James J., Jing Liu and James H. O'Keefe. 'Magnesium for the prevention and treatment of cardiovascular disease.' *Open Heart* 5, no. 2 (2018): e000775.

El Khoudary, Samar R. *et al.* 'The menopause transition and women's health at midlife: a progress report from the Study of Women's Health Across the Nation (SWAN).' *Menopause* 26, no. 10 (2019): 1213–27.

Elia, David *et al.* 'Female urine incontinence: vaginal erbium laser (VEL) effectiveness and safety.' *Hormone Molecular Biology and Clinical Investigation* 41, no. 4 (2020): 10.

Elsas, S-M *et al.* '*Passiflora incarnata* L. (passionflower) extracts elicit GABA currents in hippocampal neurons in vitro, and show anxiogenic and anticonvulsant effects in vivo, varying with extraction method.' *Phytomedicine* 17, no. 12 (2010): 940–9.

Elwishahy, Abdelrahman *et al.* '*Porphyromonas gingivalis* as a risk factor to Alzheimer's disease: a systematic review.' *Journal of Alzheimer's Disease Reports* 5, no. 1 (2021): 721–32.

'Estrogen (vaginal route).' mayoclinic.org. Accessed 8 August 2022.

European Sleep Research Society. 'European Insomnia Network.' esrs.eu. Accessed 17 August 2022.

European Society of Human Reproduction and Embryology. 'Guideline on the management of women with premature ovarian insufficiency.' December 2015. eshre.eu. Accessed 4 August 2022.

Faculty of Occupational Medicine. 'Advice on the Menopause.' fom.ac.uk. Accessed 28 October 2022.

Felix, Ashley S. *et al.* 'Intrauterine devices and endometrial cancer risk: a pooled analysis of the Epidemiology of Endometrial Cancer consortium.' *International Journal of Cancer* 136, no. 5 (2015): E410–22.

Feskanich, Diane, Walter Willett and Graham Colditz. 'Walking and leisure-time activity and risk of hip fracture in postmenopausal women.' *JAMA* 288, no. 18 (2002): 2300–6.

Finkelstein, Joel S. *et al.* 'Bone mineral density changes during the menopause transition in a multiethnic cohort of women.' *The Journal of Clinical Endocrinology and Metabolism* 93, no. 3 (2008): 861–8.

Fitzpatrick, Katherine. 'Foraging and menstruation in the Hadza of Tanzania' (doctoral thesis). University of Cambridge, 2018.

Freeman, Andrew M. and Nicholas Pennings. 'Insulin Resistance.' 4 July 2022. ncbi.nlm.nih.gov. Accessed 31 October 2022.

Freeman, Ellen W. 'Depression in the menopause transition: risks in the changing hormone milieu as observed in the general population.' *Women's Midlife Health* 1, no. 2 (2015).

Freeman, Ellen W., Mary D. Sammel and Hui Lin. 'Temporal associations of hot flashes and depression in the transition to menopause.' *Menopause* 16, no. 4 (2009): 728–34.

Gameiro, Cátia Morgado, Fatima Romão and Camil Castelo-Branco. 'Menopause and aging: changes in the immune system – a review.' *Maturitas* 67, no. 4 (2010): 316–20.

Ganesan, Ganesan Ram and Phagal Varthi Vijayaraghavan. 'Urinary N-telopeptide: the new diagnostic test for osteoporosis.' *Surgery Journal* (New York, NY) 5, no. 1 (2019): e1–e4.

Geraci, Annalisa *et al.* 'Sarcopenia and menopause: the role of estradiol.' *Frontiers in Endocrinology* 12 (2021): 682012.

Gesing, Adam. 'The thyroid gland and the process of aging.' *Thyroid Research* 8, Suppl. 1 A8 (2015).

Ghosh, Mimi, Marta Rodriguez-Garcia and Charles R. Wira. 'The immune system in menopause: pros and cons of hormone therapy.' *The Journal of Steroid Biochemistry and Molecular Biology* 142 (2014): 171–5.

Gibson, Carolyn J., Rebecca C. Thurston and Karen A. Matthews. 'Cortisol dysregulation is associated with daily diary-reported hot flashes among midlife women.' *Clinical Endocrinology* 85, no. 4 (2016): 645–51.

Gietka-Czernel, Małgorzata. 'The thyroid gland in postmenopausal women: physiology and diseases.' *Przeglad Menopauzalny = Menopause Review* 16, no. 2 (2017): 33–7.

Gold, Ellen B. 'The timing of the age at which natural menopause occurs.' *Obstetrics and Gynecology Clinics of North America* 38, no. 3 (2011): 425–40.

Gordon, Jennifer L. *et al.* 'Ovarian hormone fluctuation, neurosteroids, and HPA axis dysregulation in perimenopausal depression: a novel heuristic model.' *American Journal of Psychiatry* 172, no. 3 (2015): 227–36.

Greer, Germaine. *The Change, Women Aging and the Menopause.* New York: Alfred Knopf, 1992.

Gregorio, L. *et al.* 'Adequate dietary protein is associated with better physical performance among post-menopausal women 60–90 years.' *The Journal of Nutrition, Health & Aging* 18, no. 2 (2014): 155–60.

Grisotto, Giorgia *et al.* 'Dietary factors and onset of natural menopause: a systematic review and meta-analysis.' *Maturitas* 159 (2021): 15–32.

Guder, Christian *et al.* 'Osteoimmunology: a current update of the interplay between bone and the immune system.' *Frontiers in Immunology* 11 (2020).

Guzek, Dominika *et al.* 'Association between vitamin D supplementation and mental health in healthy adults: a systematic review.' *Journal of Clinical Medicine* 10 (2021).

Hall, Lisa *et al.* 'Meanings of menopause: cultural influences on perception and management of menopause.' *Journal of Holistic Nursing: Official Journal of the American Holistic Nurses' Association* 25, no. 2 (2007): 106–18.

Halton, Thomas L. and Frank B. Hu. 'The effects of high protein diets on thermogenesis, satiety and weight loss: a critical review. *Journal of the American College of Nutrition* 23, no. 5 (2004): 373–85.

Hamblin, Cherise Y. 'One more reason not to smoke: early menopause.' 25 October 2021. lancastergeneralhealth.org. Accessed 5 August 2022.

Hamoda H. *et al.* 'The British Menopause Society & Women's Health Concern 2020 recommendations on hormone replacement therapy in menopausal women.' *Post Reproductive Health* 26, no. 4 (2020): 181–209.

Harris, Caroline (ed.). *Daisy Network: Our Guide to Understanding Premature Ovarian Insufficiency. Tolworth*: Grosvenor House Publishing, 2021.

Harris, Caroline (ed.). *M Boldened: Menopause Conversations We All Need to Have.* Cheltenham: Flint Books, 2020.

Harrison, Fiona E. and James M. May. 'Vitamin C

function in the brain: vital role of the ascorbate transporter SVCT2.' *Free Radical Biology & Medicine* 46, no. 6 (2009): 719–30.

Harvard Medical School. 'Sugar and the brain.' hms.harvard.edu. Accessed 15 August 2022.

Harvard T.H. Chan School of Public Health. 'Carbohydrates.' hsph.harvard.edu. Accessed 15 August 2022.

Health Products Regulatory Authority. 'Aerodiol.' hpra.ie. Accessed 12 August 2022.

Health Service Executive. 'Skin cancer (melanoma).' hse.ie. Accessed 5 August 2022.

Hill K. 'The demography of menopause.' *Maturitas* 23, no. 2. (1996): 113–27.

Hoen, Sean. 'Adrenal fatigue: is it real?' 13 July 2022. endocrineweb.com. Accessed 10 August 2022.

Hollis, James. *The Midlife Passage: From Misery to Meaning in Midlife.* Toronto: Inner City, 1993.

'Home Epley maneuver.' hopkinsmedicine.org. Accessed 10 August 2022.

Hunter, Myra and Melanie Smith. 'Cognitive behaviour therapy (CBT) for menopausal symptoms.' February 2020. womens-health-concern.org. Accessed 8 August 2022.

'Hypoparathyroidism.' hopkinsmedicine.org. Accessed 5 August 2022.

International Osteoporosis Foundation. 'Factsheets.' osteoporosis.foundation. Accessed 15 August 2022.

International Osteoporosis Foundation. 'Key statistics for Europe.' osteoporosis.foundation. Accessed 15 August 2022.

Irish Heart Foundation, 'High intake of fibre in your diet reduces heart disease risk', irishheart.ie. Accessed 1 May 2022.

Irish Osteoporosis Society. 'Nutrition & bone health.' irishosteoporosis.ie. Accessed 15 August 2022.

Jackson, Philippa A. *et al.* 'Effects of saffron extract supplementation on mood, well-being, and response to a psychosocial stressor in healthy adults: a randomized, double-blind, parallel group, clinical trial.' *Frontiers in Nutrition* 7, no. 606124 (2021).

Jehan, Shazia *et al.* 'Obstructive sleep apnea: women's perspective.' *Journal of Sleep Medicine and Disorders* 3, no. 6 (2016): 1064.

Jeong, Seong-Hae. 'Benign paroxysmal positional vertigo risk factors unique to perimenopausal women.' *Frontiers in Neurology* 11 (2020).

Jones, Emma K. *et al.* 'Menopause and the influence of culture: another gap for Indigenous Australian women?.' *BMC Women's Health* 12, no. 43 (2012).

Kai, Ming Chan, Mary Anderson and Edith M. C. Lau. 'Exercise interventions: defusing the world's osteoporosis time bomb.' *Bulletin of the World Health Organization* 81, no. 11 (2003): 827–30.

Kelly, Ryan R. *et al.* 'Impacts of psychological stress on osteoporosis: clinical implications and treatment interactions.' *Frontiers in Psychiatry* 10, no. 200 (2019).

Kenealy, Brian P. *et al.* 'Neuroestradiol in the hypothalamus contributes to the regulation of gonadotropin releasing hormone release.' *Journal of Neuroscience* 33, no. 49 (2013): 19051–9.

Kim, Hyun-Kyung *et al.* 'The recent review of the genitourinary syndrome of menopause.' *Journal of Menopausal Medicine* 21, no. 2 (2015): 65–71.

Kim, Keewan *et al.* 'Dietary Intakes of vitamin b-2 (riboflavin), vitamin b-6, and vitamin b-12 and ovarian cycle function among premenopausal women.' *Journal of the Academy of Nutrition and Dietetics* 120, no. 5 (2020): 885–92.

King, H., R.E. Aubert and W.H. Herman. 'Global burden of diabetes, 1995–2025: prevalence, numerical estimates, and projections.' *Diabetes Care* 21, no. 9 (1998): 1414–31.

Kruszyńska, Aleksandra and Jadwiga Słowińska-Srzednicka. 'Anti-Müllerian hormone (AMH) as a good predictor of time of menopause.' *Przeglad Menopauzalny = Menopause Review* 16, no. 2 (2017): 47–50.

Kumano, Hiroaki. 'Osteoporosis and stress.' *Clinical Calcium* 15, no. 9 (2005): 1544–7.

La Fata, Giorgio, Peter Weber and M. Hasan Mohajeri. 'Effects of vitamin E on cognitive performance during ageing and in Alzheimer's disease.' *Nutrients* 6, no. 12 (2014): 5453–72.

Lasley, B.L., S.L. Crawford and D.S. McConnell. 'Ovarian adrenal interactions during the menopausal transition.' *Minerva Ginecologica* 65, no. 6 (2013): 641–51.

Le Couteur, D.G. *et al.* 'New horizons: dietary protein, ageing and the Okinawan ratio.' *Age and Ageing* 45, no. 4 (2016): 443–7.

Lee, Seong-Su, Kyung-do Han, Young-Hoon Joo. 'Association of perceived tinnitus with duration of hormone replacement therapy in Korean postmenopausal women: a cross-sectional study.' *BMJ Open* 7, no. 7 e013736. (2017).

Li, Cairu *et al.* 'Risk of stroke and hormone replacement therapy: a prospective cohort study. *Maturitas* 54, no. 1 (2006): 11–8.

Lim, Andrew S.P. *et al.* 'Sleep fragmentation and the risk of incident Alzheimer's disease and cognitive decline in older persons.' *Sleep* 36, no. 7 (2013): 1027–32.

Linus Pauling Institute. 'Vitamin B6'. lpi. oregonstate.edu. Accessed 28 October 2022.

Ludmann, Paula. 'I've been diagnosed with melanoma. Now what?' American Academy of Dermatology Association. aad.org. Accessed 5 August 2022.

Lund, Kamma Sundgaard *et al.* 'Efficacy of a standardised acupuncture approach for women with bothersome menopausal symptoms: a pragmatic randomised study in primary care (the ACOM study).' *BMJ* Open 9, no. 1 (2019): e023637.

Lyons, Gila. 'What is cortisol?' 13 January 2022. endocrineweb.com. Accessed 10 August 2022.

MacGregor, Anne. 'Migraine and HRT.' October 2020. womens-health-concern.org. Accessed 10 August 2022.

Maki, Pauline M. *et al.* 'Hot flashes are associated with altered brain function during a memory task.' *Menopause* 27, no. 3 (2020): 269–77.

Maltais, M.L., J. Desroches and J. Dionne. 'Changes in muscle mass and strength after menopause.' *Journal of Musculoskeletal & Neuronal Interactions* 9, no. 4 (2009): 186–97.

Mandy, Redig. 'Yams of fortune: the (uncontrolled) birth of contraceptives.' 6 September 2005. jyi.org. Accessed 12 August 2022.

Matthews, Soraya *et al. Dying and Death in Ireland: What Do We Routinely Measure, How Can We Improve?* Dublin: Irish Hospice Foundation, 2021.

Meeta, Meeta and Vishal R Tandon. 'John Studd – a tribute.' *Journal of Mid-Life Health* 12, no. 4 (2021): 251.

Melby, Melissa K. 'Chilliness: a vasomotor symptom in Japan.' *Menopause* 14, no. 4. (2007): 752–9.

'Menopause and Heart Disease.' webmd.com. Accessed 5 August 2022.

Messier, Virginie *et al.* 'Menopause and sarcopenia: a potential role for sex hormones.' *Maturitas* 68, no. 4 (2011): 331–6.

Migraine Ireland. 'Other treatment options.' migraine.ie. Accessed 10 August 2022.

Milart, Paweł *et al.* 'Selected vitamins and quality of life in menopausal women.' *Przeglad menopauzalny = Menopause review* 17, no. 4 (2018): 175–9.

Minicucci, E.M. *et al.* 'Assessing the impact of menopause on salivary flow and xerostomia.' *Australian Dental Journal* 58, no. 2 (2013): 230–4.

Mnif, Wissem *et al.* 'Effect of endocrine disruptor pesticides: a review.' *International Journal of Environmental Research and Public Health* 8, no. 6 (2011): 2265–303.

Morimoto, Yukiko *et al.* 'Urinary estrogen metabolites during a randomized soy trial.' *Nutrition and Cancer* 64, no. 2 (2012): 307–14.

Morris, Danielle *et al.* 'Familial concordance for age at natural menopause: results from the Breakthrough Generations Study.' *Menopause* 18, no. 9 (2011): 956–61.

Mosconi, Lisa. *The XX Brain*. London: Allen and Unwin, 2020.

Mosconi, Lisa *et al.* 'Menopause impacts human brain structure, connectivity, energy metabolism, and amyloid-beta deposition.' *Scientific Reports 11*, no. 1 *(2021).*

Mukherjee, Dr Annice. *The Complete Guide to the Menopause.* London: Vermilion, 2021.

Muscat Baron, Yves. 'A history of the menopause'. University of Malta Medical School: The Department of Obstetrics and Gynaecology, Faculty of Medicine and Surgery, 2012.

Nanda, K. *et al.* 'Hormone replacement therapy and the risk of colorectal cancer: a meta-analysis.' *Obstetrics and Gynecology* 93,no. 5 Pt. 2 (1999): 880–8.

Nasiadek, Marzenna *et al.* 'The role of zinc in selected female reproductive system disorders.' *Nutrients* 12, no. 8 (2020): 2464.

National Center for Complementary and Integrative Health. 'Acupuncture, as practiced in clinical settings, may significantly improve menopause-related symptoms.' 18 March 2016. nccih.nih.gov. Accessed 8 August 2022.

National Institute for Health and Care Excellence. 'Menopause: diagnosis and management.' 12 November 2015. nice.org.uk. Accessed 10 August 2022.

National Institute for Health and Care Research. 'Risk of breast cancer with HRT depends on therapy type and duration.' 20 December 2021. evidence.nihr.ac.uk. Accessed 12 August 2022.

National Institute for Occupational Safety and Health. 'Sleep pressure: homeostatic sleep drive.' cdc.gov. Accessed 17 August 2022.

National Institute of Child Health and Human Development. 'Bone loss in Depo-Provera users largely reversible.' 6 September 2002. nichd.nih.gov. Accessed 15 August 2022.

National Institutes of Health. 'How too little potassium may contribute to cardiovascular disease.' 24 October 2017. nih.gov. Accessed 30 October 2022.

National Library of Medicine, 'Four grams of glucose', ncbi.nlm.nih.gov. Accessed 1 May 2022.

National Library of Medicine, 'Milk thistle', ncbi.nlm.nih.gov. Accessed 30 October 2022.

National Library of Medicine, 'Postmenopausal cognitive changes and androgen levels in the context of apolipoprotein E polymorphism', ncbi.nlm.nih.gov. Accessed February 2022.

Nechuta, Sarah J. *et al.* 'Soy food intake after diagnosis of breast cancer and survival: an in-depth analysis of combined evidence from cohort studies of US and Chinese women.' *The American Journal of Clinical Nutrition* 96, no. 1 (2012): 123–32.

'Neurosteroids.' sciencedirect.com. Accessed 5 August 2022.

Newson, Louise *et al.* 'Position statement for management of genitourinary syndrome of the menopause (GSM).' bssm.org.uk. Accessed 8 August 2022.

Newson, Louise R. 'Best practice for HRT: unpicking the evidence.' *The British Journal of General Practice: The Journal of the Royal College of General Practitioners* 66, no. 653 (2016): 597–8.

Nguyen, Thuy Trang *et al.* 'Type 3 diabetes and its role implications in Alzheimer's disease.' *International Journal of Molecular Sciences* 21, no. 9 (2020): 3165.

NHS Inform. 'Early and premature menopause.' nhsinform.scot. Accessed 15 August 2022.

NIH National Institute on Aging. 'Memory, forgetfulness, and aging: what's normal and what's not?' nia.nih.gov. Accessed 15 August 2022.

North American Menopause Society 2017 Hormone Therapy Position Statement Advisory Panel. 'The 2017 hormone therapy position statement of the North American Menopause Society.' *Menopause* (New York, NY) 24, no. 7 (2017): 728–53.

North American Menopause Society. 'Depression & menopause.' menopause.org. Accessed 10 August 2022.

North American Menopause Society. 'Hot flashes impair memory performance: new study suggests hot flashes may alter hippocampal and prefrontal cortex function to decrease verbal memory.' sciencedaily.com. Accessed 8 August 2022.

North American Menopause Society. 'Natural remedies for hot flashes.' menopause.org. Accessed 5 August 2022.

Nutt, David, Sue Wilson and Louise Paterson. 'Sleep disorders as core symptoms of depression.' *Dialogues in Clinical Neuroscience* 10, no. 3 (2008): 329–36.

Ogun, Oluwaseye Ayoola *et al.* 'Menopause and benign paroxysmal positional vertigo.' *Menopause* 21, no. 8 (2014): 886–9.

Olson, Christopher R. and Claudio V. Mello. 'Significance of vitamin A to brain function, behavior and learning.' *Molecular Nutrition & Food Research* 54, no. 4 (2010): 489–95.

O'Reilly, Barry. 'Vaginal erbium laser for SUI: a prospective multicentre randomized placebo-controlled trial to evaluate efficacy and safety of non-ablative Er:YAG laser for treatment of stress urinary incontinence (SUI).' Webinar from ICS 2021 Melbourne Online. ics.org.

'Ospemifene tablet – uses, side effects, and more.' webmd.com. Accessed 8 August 2022.

Pacheco, Danielle. 'Menopause and sleep.' 6 May 2022. sleepfoundation.org. Accessed 17 August 2022.

Pacheco, Danielle. 'What's the best time of day to exercise for sleep?' 5 April 2022. sleepfoundation.org. Accessed 17 August 2022.

Panay, Nick and Anna Fenton. 'Bioidentical hormones: what is all the hype about?.' *Climacteric: the Journal of the International Menopause Society* 13, no. 1 (2010): 1–3.

Panay, Nick. 'Testosterone replacement in menopause.' May 2022. thebms.org.uk. Accessed 8 August 2022.

Panay, Nick *et al.* 'Premature ovarian insufficiency: an International Menopause Society white paper.' October 2020. imsociety.org. Accessed 12 August 2022.

Peck, Travis, Leslie Olsakovsky and Shruti Aggarwal. 'Dry eye syndrome in menopause and perimenopausal age group.' *Journal of Mid-Life Health* 8, no. 2 (2017): 51–4.

Penckofer, Sue *et al.* 'Vitamin D and depression: where is all the sunshine?.' *Issues in Mental Health Nursing* 31, no. 6 (2010): 385–93.

Perez, Caroline Criado. *Invisible Women: Exposing Data Bias in a World Designed for Men.* London: Vintage, 2019.

'Periodic limb movement disorder (PLMD) in adults.' my.clevelandclinic.org. Accessed 17 August 2022.

'Phenytoin (oral route).' mayoclinic.org. Accessed 12 August 2022.

'Phenytoin.' nhs.uk. Accessed 12 August 2022.

Pikul, Corrie. 'Why are Black Americans twice as likely to have Alzheimer's or other dementias as white Americans?' *Boston Globe*, 29 October 2020.

Pollycove, Ricki, Frederick Naftolin and James A. Simon. 'The evolutionary origin and significance of menopause.' *Menopause* 18, no. 3 (2011): 336–42.

Pope, Alexandra and Sjanie Hugo Wurlitzer. *Wild Power.* London: Hay House UK, 2017.

'Postmenopausal hormone therapy associated with higher risk of hearing loss.' 10 May 2017. womens-health-concern.org. Accessed 10 August 2022.

'Prasterone (dehydroepiandrosterone, DHEA) vaginal.' peacehealth.org. Accessed 8 August 2022.

Price, Charles T., Joshua R Langford and Frank A. Liporace. 'Essential nutrients for bone health and a review of their availability in the average North American diet.' *The Open Orthopaedics Journal* 6 (2012): 143–9.

Price, Charles T., Kenneth J. Koval and Joshua R. Langford. 'Silicon: a review of its potential role in the prevention and treatment of postmenopausal osteoporosis.' *International Journal of Endocrinology* 2013 (2013): 316783.

Prior, Dr Jerilynn. *Estrogen's Storm Season: Stories of Perimenopause.* Vancouver: Centre for Menstrual Cycle and Ovulation Research, 2005.

Rahman, Aneela, Eva Schelbaum *et al.* 'Sex-driven modifiers of Alzheimer risk: a multimodality brain imaging study.' Neurology 95, no. 2 (2020): e166-e178.

Rahman, Aneela, Hande Jackson *et al.* 'Sex and gender driven modifiers of Alzheimer's: the role for estrogenic control across age, race, medical, and lifestyle risks.' *Frontiers in Aging Neuroscience* 11, no. 315 (2019).

Rapaport, Lisa. 'Culture may influence how women experience menopause.' 5 June 2015. reuters.com. Accessed 5 August 2022.

Reddy, Doodipala Samba. 'Neurosteroids: endogenous role in the human brain and therapeutic potentials.' *Progress in Brain Research*, 186 (2010): 113–37.

Rees Margaret *et al.* 'Global consensus recommendations on menopause in the workplace: a European Menopause and Andropause Society (EMAS) position statement.' *Maturitas* 151 (2021): 55–62.

Reese, I. 'Nutrition therapy for adverse reactions to histamine in food and beverages.' *Allergol Select* 2, no. 1 (2018): 56–61.

Reginster, Jean-Yves *et al.* 'Osteoporosis and sarcopenia: two diseases or one?' *Current Opinion in Clinical Nutrition and Metabolic Care* 19, no. 1 (2016): 31–6.

Riemann, Dieter, Chiara Baglioni *et al.* 'European guideline for the diagnosis and treatment of insomnia.' *Journal of Sleep Research* 26, no. 6 (2017): 675–700.

Roth, Thomas. 'Insomnia: definition, prevalence, etiology, and consequences.' *Journal of Clinical Sleep Medicine* 3, no. 5 Suppl. *(2007)*: S7–10.

Rozen, T.D. *et al.* 'Open label trial of coenzyme Q10 as a migraine preventive.' Cephalalgia: *An International Journal of Headache* 22, no. 2 (2002): 137–41.

Santen, Richard J. and Evan Simpson. 'History of estrogen: its purification, structure, synthesis, biologic actions, and clinical applications.' *Endocrinology* 160, no. 3 (2019): 605–25.

Scavello, Irene *et al.* 'Sexual health in menopause.' *Medicina* (Kaunas) 55, no. 9 (2019): 559.

Schelbaum, Eva *et al.* 'Association of reproductive history with brain MRI biomarkers of dementia risk in midlife.' *Neurology* 97, no. 23 (2021): e2328-e2339.

Schwalfenberg, Gerry Kurt. 'Vitamins K1 and K2: the emerging group of vitamins required for human health.' *Journal of Nutrition and Metabolism* 2017 (2017): 6254836.

Seaborg, Eric. 'Underdiagnosed & undertreated: the mysteries of genitourinary syndrome of menopause.' December 2016. endocrinenews. endocrine.org. Accessed 8 August 2022.

Shanmugan, Sheila and C. Neill Epperson. 'Estrogen and the prefrontal cortex: towards a new understanding of estrogen's effects on executive functions in the menopause transition.' *Human Brain Mapping* 35, no. 3 (2014): 847–65.

Shellenbarger, Sue. *The Breaking Point: How Today's Women Are Navigating Midlife Crisis.* New York: Henry Holt & Company, 2005.

Short, Dr Hannah and Dr Mandy Leonhardt. *The Complete Guide to POI and Early Menopause.* London: Sheldon Press, 2022.

Slopien, R. *et al.* 'Climacteric symptoms are related to thyroid status in euthyroid menopausal women.' *Journal of Endocrinological Investigation* 43, no. 1 (2020): 75–80.

Statista Research Department. 'Number of hysterectomies conducted in Ireland 2006–2020.' 22 July 2022. statista.com. Accessed 5 August 2022.

Stein, Murray. *In Midlife: A Jungian Perspective.* Dallas: Spring Publications, 1983.

Stevenson, John. 'Osteoporosis: bone health following the menopause.' womens-health-concern.org. Accessed 15 August 2022.

Stewart, Donna E. 'Menopause in highland Guatemala Mayan women.' *Maturitas* 44, no. 4 (2003): 293–7.

Stirrat, Siofra, Maire McCallion and Azura Youell. 'An Evaluation of the Green Prescription Programme in County Donegal 2013.' hse.ie. Accessed 10 August 2022.

Stolberg, Michael. 'A woman's hell? Medical perceptions of menopause in preindustrial Europe.' *Bulletin of the History of Medicine* 73, no. 3 (1999): 404–28.

Studd, John and Rossella E. Nappi. 'Reproductive

depression and the response to estrogen therapy.' studd.co.uk. Accessed 10 August 2022.

Studd, John and Rossella E. Nappi. 'Reproductive depression.' *Gynecological Endocrinology: The Official Journal of the International Society of Gynecological Endocrinology* 28 Suppl. 1 (2012): 42–5.

Studd, John. 'Oestrogen treatment for depression in women – are psychiatrists missing something?' 5 February 2010. studd.co.uk. Accessed 10 August 2022.

Sydora, Beate C. *et al.* 'Menopause experience in First Nations women and initiatives for menopause symptom awareness: a community-based participatory research approach.' *BMC Women's Health* 21, no. 179 (2021).

Takacs, Peter *et al.* 'Zinc-containing vaginal moisturizer gel improves postmenopausal vulvovaginal symptoms: a pilot study.' *Journal of Menopausal Medicine* 25, no. 1 (2019): 63–8.

'Target heart rate calculator.' active.com. Accessed 10 August 2022.

Tawwab, Nedra Glover. *Set Boundaries, Find Peace.* New York: Penguin, 2021.

Temple, Robert K.G. and Joseph Needham. *The Genius of China: 3,000 Years of Science, Discovery, and Invention.* New York: Simon and Schuster, 1986.

Thebe, Amanda. *Menopocalypse.* Vancouver: Greystone Books, 2020.

Thurston, Rebecca C. and Hadine Joffe. 'Vasomotor symptoms and menopause: findings from the Study of Women's Health across the Nation.' *Obstetrics and Gynecology Clinics of North America* 38, no. 3 (2011): 489–501.

Tilt, E.J. 'On the management of women at, and after the cessation of, menstruation.' *Provincial Medical and Surgical Journal (1844–1852)* 15, no. 20 (1851): 545–8.

Timur, Sermin and Nevin Hotun Sahin. 'The prevalence of depression symptoms and influencing factors among perimenopausal and postmenopausal women.' *Menopause* 17, no. 3 (2010): 545–51.

Trinity College Dublin. 'New research reveals where and how people die in Ireland.' 25 November 2021. tcd.ie. Accessed 4 August 2022.

Tsutsui, Kazuyoshi, Shogo Haraguchi. *Handbook of Hormones: Comparative Endocrinology for Basic and Clinical Research.* Oxford: Academic Press, 2015.

University of California – San Francisco. 'When it comes to sleep, it's quality over quantity.' 15 March 2022. sciencedaily.com. Accessed 27 October 2022.

University of Exeter. 'New evidence of menopause in killer whales.' 20 July 2021. sciencedaily. com. Accessed 28 July 2022.

University of Oxford. 'Million Women Study: data sharing.' millionwomenstudy.org. Accessed 12 August 2022.

University of Oxford. 'The million women study.' web.archive.org. Accessed 12 August 2022.

van de Straat, Vera, and Piet Bracke. 'How well does Europe sleep? A cross-national study of sleep problems in European older adults.' *International Journal of Public Health* 60, no. 6 (2015): 643–50.

van der Kolk, Bessel. *The Body Keeps the Score: Mind, Brain and Body in the Transformation of Trauma.* London: Penguin Books, 2014.

Van Trotsenburg, Mick and Maria Cristina Meriggiola. 'Transgender and menopause.' International Menopause Society. 2 September 2021. Webinar, YouTube.

Velez, Adriana. 'Menopause is different for women of color.' 10 March 2021. endocrineweb.com. Accessed 5 August 2022.

Vivian-Taylor, Josephine and Martha Hickey. 'Menopause and depression: is there a link?' *Maturitas* 79, no. 2 (2014): 142–6.

Volpi, Elena *et al.* 'Muscle tissue changes with aging.' Current Opinion in Clinical Nutrition and Metabolic Care 7, no. 4 (2004): 405–10.

Walker, Dr Matthew. *Why We Sleep.* London: Penguin Books, 2017.

Wang, Chao-Yung. 'Circadian rhythm, exercise, and heart.' *Acta Cardiologica Sinica* 33, no. 5 (2017): 539–41.

Ward, Mark, Richard Layte and Rose Anne Kenny. *Loneliness, Social Isolation, and Their Discordance among Older Adults: Findings from The Irish Longitudinal Study on Ageing* (TILDA). Trinity College Dublin, 2019.

Whiteley, Jennifer *et al.* 'The impact of menopausal symptoms on quality of life, productivity, and economic outcomes.' *Journal of Women's Health* 22, no. 11 (2013): 983–90.

Wójcik, Oktawia P. *et al.* 'The potential protective effects of taurine on coronary heart disease.' *Atherosclerosis* 208, no. 1 (2010): 19–25.

Women's Health Concern. 'Testosterone for women.' February 2022. womens-health-concern.org. Accessed 28 October 2022.

Woodyard, Catherine. 'Exploring the therapeutic effects of yoga and its ability to increase quality of life.' *International Journal of Yoga* 4, no. 2 (2011): 49–54.

World Health Organization. '10 facts on gender and tobacco.' who.int. Accessed 5 August 2022.

Worsley, Robin *et al.* 'Prevalence and predictors of low sexual desire, sexually related personal distress, and hypoactive sexual desire dysfunction in a community-based sample of midlife women.' *The Journal of Sexual Medicine* 14, no. 5 (2017): 675–86.

Wu, A. *et al.* 'Epidemiology of soy exposures and breast cancer risk.' *British Journal of Cancer* 98 (2008): 9–14.

Yang, Hee Jung, Pae Sun Suh, Soo Jeong Kim, and Soon Young Lee. 'Effects of smoking on menopausal age: results from the Korea National Health and Nutrition Examination Survey, 2007 to 2012.' *Journal of Preventive Medicine and Public Health = Yebang Uihakhoe Chi 48*, no. 4 (2015): 216–24.

Zakrzewska, Joanna, and John A.G. Buchanan. 'Burning mouth syndrome.' *BMJ Clinical Evidence* (2016): 1301.

Zeleke, Berihun. 'Vasomotor and Sexual Symptoms in Community-Dwelling Older Australian Women.' *Fertility and Sterility* 105, no. 1 (2015): 149–55.

Ziaei, S., A. Kazemnejad and M. Zareai. 'The effect of vitamin E on hot flashes in menopausal women.' *Gynecologic and Obstetric Investigation* 64, no. 4 (2007): 204–7.

Zierau, Oliver, Ana C. Zenclussen and Federico Jensen. 'Role of female sex hormones, estradiol and progesterone, in mast cell behavior.' *Frontiers in Immunology* 3 (2012).

Zuelsdorff, Megan *et al.* 'Stressful life events and racial disparities in cognition among middle-aged and older adults.' *Journal of Alzheimer's Disease* 73, no. 2 (2020): 671–82.

Acknowledgements

'**I** just don't feel like myself any more.' If there was a prompt to write this book, it is that phrase over and over again from the countless women I have spoken with. Writing a book on menopause is not an individual process, but a community effort, so heartfelt thanks to the many women who have shared with me over the last number of years their own menopause experiences, and especially to those whose stories feature in this book. To those I have met in person, at the summits, through workplaces or virtually, your smiles made all the difference.

Thank you to the lovely warm, supportive Wellness Warrior community, to all of you on social media and on email who have followed this journey with me – your incredible support, laughs and encouragement all the way mean so much to me.

To the hundreds of workplaces that have invited me in and supported menopause – you are making an impact, and your support not only helps the person going through menopause but everyone in that person's life.

A special thanks to my editor, Emma Dunne, who shared my passion in editing this book and is an absolute joy to work with. Thanks to all the team at The O'Brien Press – it has been a great experience working with you. Thanks also to Camilla Shestopal for her guidance in the world of writing.

To the fellow menopause enthusiasts in my life who have helped me in one way or another with this book: Sarah Brereton, Tom Coleman, Mary Rose Devereux, Mary Lynn, Dr Brenda Moran, Michele O'Brien, Professor Moira O'Brien, Roisin O'Kelly, Alva O Sullivan, Dr Caoimhe Ryan, Dr Hannah Short, Amanda Thebe, Maeve Whelan, Lavinia Winch. For anyone in Waterford, Teresa Murphy of Nature's Remedies is a local treasure and a hero of mine.

A special word of thanks to Diane Danzebrink, of #MakeMenopauseMatter, for all her support in various aspects of this book and in the rollercoaster ride that is menopause awareness.

Huge thanks to the team behind the Menopause Success Summit – we started out to help women and I believe we are doing our small part here. Fiona and Aisling Kelly, the calmest duo ever, thank you.

I had the great pleasure of meeting the dynamic duo of Frank Prendergast and Marci Corbett several years ago and have never looked back. Thank you for being constant supporters and advocates of my passion for menopause and for the many shared laughs along the way.

Throughout my life I have been blessed with the most incredible people, friends who have shared all life's up and downs and supported me in a million ways in writing this book. To Marguerite Kervick for being a constant friend and always the best craic. Hormones start way back in puberty – Sinead Byrne and Anita Carey, thanks for supporting my menopause journey which began back then. To my college gang, Kate Cullen, Anne Flood, Anne Hill, Sinead McGorrian and Amanda Madden – you were there from the start and that's not Copenhagen! Tanya Cunningham and Fiona Mahon – parenting and writing were made easier with you both on the ride.

Movement is a key part of my life and my running family are the backbone – you ran with me through all these pages and I am so grateful for your support, review of these pages, laughs and endless coffees along the way. The endurance athletes, legends and nutters that you are, you make me smile even on those hills! To Robyn and Anna at the Windowbox for the best power salad in Dublin.

A special mention to all my friends and work colleagues from my investment banking days – my chapter there brought me here. It was a privilege to work with you all and to have made such great lifelong friendships – too many to name, but you know who you are.

To my family and my cousins for support on the sidelines and childhood memories. Tony, Teresa, Dervla, Brian, Rob and Art, my Rathfarnham clan, for so much. Growing up with cousins born within months of each other was the best – Harry, Mark, Paul and Valerie, I am glad I educated you all on menopause! I have been so lucky to have had support not just in Ireland but also from abroad. I know no stronger women than my beautiful cousins the Tallent sisters: Mary, Therese, Gabriel and Pia, thank you for all your lovely messages along the way. Thanks to Lisa, Paul and Theo for the countless cups of tea, laughs and chats and support in writing this book. To my in-laws, who have always made me feel part of the family. And to John Cashin for endless chocolate pies, walks and support.

To my parents who started me on this crazy journey of life and taught me so much along the way, from my love of trees to my appreciation of kindness.

My big sister, Vivienne O'Keeffe, you have been there since I was a nipper and you have been the best supporter of Wellness Warrior from the start. Thank you for teaching me so much about life and encouraging me out of my comfort zone. Here's to many more hikes together.

Finally, menopause is only one side of my life – the other is my boys. Life is never dull. To Charlie for always bringing your humour, to Harry for the best playlist ever and to Luke for dancing, writing and adding all forms of art to our lives. To Tom for bringing the music into my life – thank you for holding quiet when the narkiness struck, for picking up the slack when deadlines hit and for being in my corner. And of course the essential ingredient, as the boys always remind me: Joy, our dog, the queen of the house, featured in many social media videos and the best company on many a hike in Marley and Cruagh. My life would be far too boring without you all in it – love you around all the football pitches, zoos and F1 tracks, Flores Island and beyond.

Big hugs,
Catherine

Index